COLUMBIA COLLEGE

3 2711 00016 5092

D1786413

DISCARD

ENTERED OCT 1 8 1993

TEACHING PERSONALITY WITH GRACEFULNESS

The Transmission of Japanese Cultural Values Through Japanese Dance Theatre

Barbara Sellers-Young
Department of Dramatic Art
University of California, Davis

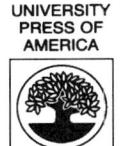

UNIVERSITY
PRESS OF
AMERICA

Lanham • New York • London

Copyright © 1993 by
University Press of America®, Inc.
4720 Boston Way
Lanham, Maryland 20706

3 Henrietta Street
London WC2E 8LU England

All rights reserved
Printed in the United States of America
British Cataloging in Publication Information Available

Library of Congress Cataloging-in-Publication Data

Sellers-Young, Barbara.
Teaching personality with gracefulness : the transmission of
Japanese cultural values through Japanese dance theatre /
by Barbara Sellers-Young.
p. cm.
Includes bibliographical references and index.
1. Dancing—Japan—Study and teaching. 2. Japan—Social life and customs—Study and teaching—Northwest, Pacific. 3. Fujima, Kanriye. I. Title.
GV1695.S45   1993   793.31952—dc20   92–41782 CIP

ISBN 0-8191-9014-4 (cloth : alk. paper)
ISBN 0-8191-9015-2 (pbk. : alk. paper)

```
793.31952 S467t

Sellers-Young, Barbara.

Teaching personality with
gracefulness
```

 The paper used in this publication meets the minimum requirements of American National Standard for Information Sciences—Permanence of Paper for Printed Library Materials, ANSI Z39.48–1984.

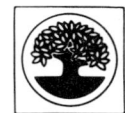

To

Kanriye Fujima and all the immigrant
women artists who have created a new
life in the United States.

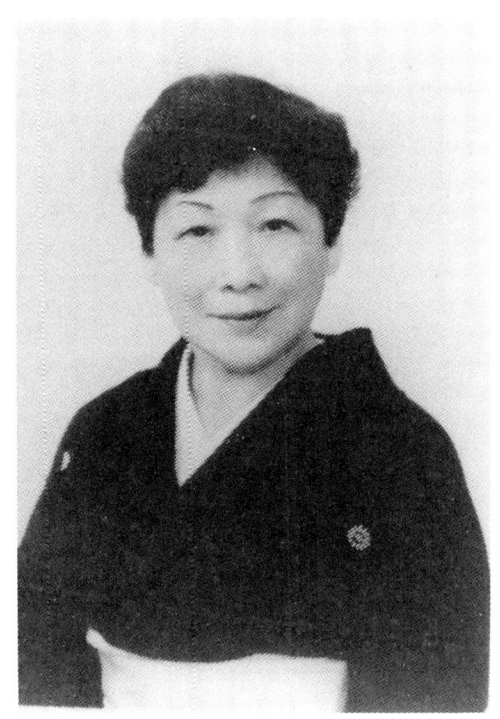

Kanriye Fujima

ACKNOWLEDGEMENTS

This manuscript would not have been possible without the help and guidance of many different people. Jonah Salz and the Traditional Theatre Training Program were instrumental in providing the experience that provided the initial introduction to Japanese theatre. The Center for the Study of Women in Society at the University of Oregon supported the research with a fieldwork grant. Robert Barton was responsible for pointing me in the direction of becoming a theatre movement specialist. Beverly Jones was a wonderful listener and guide during the fieldwork process. Larry Kominz read many different drafts of the manuscript and served as a thoughtful collaborator in the area of Japanese theatre and advisor on Japanese language and terminology. Charlene Gates was very helpful in directing the shape of the manuscript in its early stages. Philip Young made insightful contributions to my understanding of the relationship between theatre and culture. Sara Townsend made very useful editorial comments. Lia Scott's graphics helped enormously to elucidate the text. Rebecca and Roy Conant have provided constant support at every stage of the project from fieldwork to final publication. Vicki Kobayashi generously shared her home and asked extremely intelligent questions. Barbara Uyesugi was constantly encouraging of my study of *nihon buyo*. The members of Fujinami-kai gave generously of their time. Kanriye Fujima gave me a life time gift with her insistence on my becoming a student.

Barbara Sellers-Young
Davis, California
October 1992

CONTENTS

	Page
PREFACE	xiii

CHAPTER

I.	BECOMING A STUDENT	1
II.	KANRIYE FUJIMA'S LIFE AND TRADITIONAL JAPANESE DANCE THEATRE	15
III.	THE MOVEMENT AND ITS AESTHETIC BASE	35
IV.	THE STUDENTS	55
V.	THE STUDIO: THE PROCESS OF TEACHING	69
VI.	THE PERFORMANCE ELEMENTS	95
VII.	CONTEXTS OF PERFORMANCE	121
VIII.	NIHON BUYO: FROM JAPAN TO THE PACIFIC NORTHWEST	145

APPENDICES

| A. | THE DANCES AND PROGRAM NOTES OF FUJINAMI-KAI | 171 |
| B. | THE TEN MOST TAUGHT DANCES IN EACH AGE CATEGORY | 209 |

REFERENCES	211
INDEX	221

LIST OF ILLUSTRATIONS

CHART 5-A: QUALITIES OF PERSONALITY WITH GRACEFULNESS	91

CHART 8-A: A FLOW CHART OF THE RELATIONSHIPS BETWEEN KANRIYE FUJIMA AND CONTEXTS OF JAPAN AND THE UNITED STATES	147
CHART 8-B: QUALITIES OF PERSONALITY WITH GRACEFULNESS ACQUIRED FROM DIFFERENT ASPECTS OF TRAINING	151
CHART 8-C: THE RELATIONSHIP BETWEEN THE NATORI, THE COMMUNITIES, AND THE PERFORMANCE CONTEXT	159
FIGURE 3-A: WESTERN TRAINED DANCER	36
FIGURE 3-B: JAPANESE TRAINED DANCER	36
FIGURE 3-C: ONNAGATA POSE	41
FIGURE 3-D: ONNAGATA POSE	42
FIGURE 3-E: ARAGOTO POSE	43
FIGURE 3-F: ARAGOTO POSE	44
FIGURE 6-A: DIANE HINATSU IN FUJI MUSUME	111
FIGURE 6-B: BARBARA UYESUGI IN UKIYO DOJOJI	112
FIGURE 6-C: AMANDA LAU IN MAIKO	113
FIGURE 6-D: MIYOKO STROUP IN MASK PORTION OF OHARAME	114
FIGURE 6-E: MIYOKO STROUP IN OHARAME	115
FIGURE 6-F: KRISTINA KORA IN KAGUYAHIME	116
FIGURE 6-G: ELISE OKAZAKI AND ANGELA KORA IN URESHII HINAMATSURI	117
FIGURE 6-H: KRISTINA KORA AND AMANDA LAU IN NOZAKI KOUTA	118
FIGURE 7-A: OBON PERFORMANCE SPACE	132
TABLE 7-A: TABLE OF PERFORMANCES	140

PREFACE

This is a study of how Kanriye Fujima translates the traditional theatre training she received in Japan to the cultural milieu of the Pacific Northwest. In the text, I review her life from her birth in Japan to the redevelopment of her life in the United States. I describe the process of teaching, the contexts of performances, and the themes and images associated with the dance theatre pieces. This review of her life and work provides insight into how a person raised in one culture is able to transmit the essentials of a theatre form to other groups of people whose social backgrounds are different. It also illustrates the influence the theatre form has on the lives of the students.

The primary theme of this book is 'personality with gracefulness.' Each chapter either directly or indirectly refers to this concept from a different point of view, ranging from its association with traditional training systems in Japan to the construction of Kanriye Fujima's life and teaching in the United States, and to the function of this concept within the lives of Kanriye Fujima's students.

There are, throughout the book and in Appendix A, many references to *nihon buyo* pieces. Because the setting of this story is an American community, I have followed the spelling of the dances as they have appeared in Fujinami-kai programs. In some cases, the spellings used here differ from those to be found in the scholarly literature. I have not included *kanji* translations because, with rare exceptions, the programs are not in *kanji*. Within the book, I have written Japanese names, whether representing people from Japan or the United States, using the custom followed in the United States of the family name last, as in Kanriye Fujima, rather than Japanese custom of the family name first, as in Fujima Kanriye. This is the style used by the *nihon buyo* schools overseen by Kanriye Fujima.

CHAPTER I

BECOMING A STUDENT

On a pleasantly warm spring day in March of 1986 I drove from my home in Eugene to a house in northeast Portland to study *nihon buyo*[1] with a teacher of the Fujima school of Japan. As I drove down the freeway, I found I was becoming increasingly concerned about committing some unpardonable breach of Japanese etiquette. Two months spent in Japan in 1985 studying *nihon buyo* had taught me the basic verbal and nonverbal behavior required for taking a lesson. However, I knew the behavior I had learned in that short time was not yet ingrained and that I had not mastered the complex etiquette used by the Japanese in a formal student-teacher relationship. I was also certain that the many books I had read on Japanese customs had not replaced my European American upbringing in a small town in Oregon. Nervously I walked down the stairs to the basement studio reminding myself that, even though the other students might not share my ethnic heritage, the other students and I were all products of the American educational system. As I approached the door of the basement studio, I could hear the twang of a *shamisen* (Japanese three-stringed instrument) and a Japanese woman's voice in heavily accented English telling someone to "Look at mommy and then look at the umbrella." Following the instructions posted next to the closed door, I removed my shoes and set them adjacent to those of the other students.[2] Then I took a deep breath and entered the room.

A young girl about five years of age stood in the middle of a slightly raised wooden floor that covered most of the surface of the room. A tiny woman dressed in a blue patterned *kimono* (a floor length garment with wide sleeves) and matching *obi* (sash tied around the center of the *kimono*) sat in a straight backed wooden chair next to a tape recorder. As the Japanese music poured forth from the tape recorder, the woman, using a series of hand gestures, guided the little girl through a short *nihon buyo* piece. The little girl's attention was completely focused on the woman in front of her as she moved with a combination of ease and awkwardness from one phrase of music to the next. On the edge of the wooden floor just inside the door several women sat on two low-cushioned couches, their attention focused on the teacher and the young girl. I quickly sat on the floor in the formal Japanese style called *seiza* (knees and feet tucked under the body), trying to be as inconspicuous as possible.

A few minutes later the young girl completed her lesson. Barbara Uyesugi, the Japanese American head of Kanriye Fujima's Portland based school, Fujinami-kai, came and introduced herself to me. Indicating I should follow her, she led me to the woman who had been directing the lesson, Kanriye Fujima, whom she called Sensei (teacher).[3] While I tried to determine the best possible etiquette by watching Barbara's general demeanor, Kanriye Fujima inquired about the dance pieces I had studied while I was in Japan. I explained that my study in Japan had been very brief and I had only learned one dance piece. In a voice filled with encouragement she said "I am certain you will be a good student," and immediately sent me to change into my *yukata* (cotton practice *kimono*) so we could begin my lesson.

After struggling for several minutes to get my *obi* tied correctly, I gave up and came out of the bathroom with the *obi* in my hand. Kanriye Fujima, with a patient smile, took the *obi* and demonstrated how to put it on correctly. In the process of tying the *obi* around my waist, she also rearranged my *yukata*. The *yukata* appropriately wrapped, I knelt in *seiza* in the center of the wooden floor, giving the polite Japanese phrase "*onegai shimasu*," which thanks the teacher in advance for being willing to teach. During the next half-hour, I attempted to absorb the movement Kanriye was teaching, both by following her body in front of me and her reflection in the full-length mirrors on the wall behind the tape recorder. My study of *nihon buyo* had begun.

The Process of Field Research

As Georges and Jones so thoroughly document in their book, *People Studying People*, field work has always been an extended dialogue between the ethnographer and the people with whom he/she is working. Mary Sheridan and Janet Salaff (1984), in their discussion of a group study on the lives of Chinese women also point out the amorphous nature of the ethnographic relationship:

> Most of our authors followed their subjects into several different environments and among many different people, either physically or verbally. The authors noted the social interaction of the women and the roles they assumed in different contexts. The authors also became aware of themselves as a factor in the environment; if the setting of the interactions changed, the interviewer herself sometimes assumed a different role. This method is fluid, many faceted, and distinct from the single neutral or controlled environment interview paradigm adapted from laboratory science. (p. 10)

Fieldwork for both interviewer and informant initiates a complex relationship which evolves over time during a continuing series of confrontations and compromises:

> Fieldwork requiring people to study other people at first hand, however, entails much more than merely knowing what to observe and how to record, process and present it. The field worker must explain his or her presence and purpose to others, gain their confidence and cooperation, and develop and maintain mutually acceptable relationships. These requirements create dilemmas, produce confrontations, demand clarifications and compromises, and evoke reflections and introspection that one can neither fully anticipate nor prepare for in advance. Worthwhile projects may fail. Research strategies frequently must be modified or abandoned as researchers and subjects interact. Unexpected opportunities, fruitful leads, and important insights can blossom as fieldwork develops. (Georges and Jones, 1980, p. 2)

My original intention in studying the *nihon buyo* dance theatre form was to investigate the life of noted teacher Kanriye Fujima and the methods she uses to teach a Japanese art form to students in three Pacific Northwest communities. I had planned to accomplish this through observation of lessons and a series of extended interviews. But as I proceeded with the study and the lessons I found that it was not I, the ethnographer, directing the study of a subject, but rather Kanriye Fujima who directed the flow of perceived information; in fact, it was she who consciously guided the shape of the material. In so doing, she communicated to me as an individual, as well as an ethnographer, the concept she perceived as being the focus of her life's work as a teacher: 'personality with gracefulness.'

This study is based primarily on my experiences for two and one-half years as a participating member of the Portland-based Fujinami-kai, and for seven months as a resident of Ontario, Oregon, where Kanriye Fujima makes her permanent home.[4] Much of my initial behavior as a researcher was not at all congruent, from Kanriye Fujima's perspective, to that of a student. At first, I failed from her point of view to demonstrate enough respect for my teacher and the artistic tradition she represented. As an enthusiastic field worker, I asked too many questions about the dance theatre pieces, about how she taught in Japan in comparison to the United States, and about her personal life. When the answers were not forthcoming, I sometimes, without realizing it, committed a tremendous breach of etiquette by creating a confrontation with more questions. By attempting to control the kind of data I was collecting, I failed--from her point of view--to understand my proper position as a student and to convey the proper humility and respect for my teacher that this role entailed. Kanriye Fujima, with a combination of gentleness and determination, fulfilled those of my requests that were appropriate within the traditional system and quietly ignored those she felt were not. In this process she was aided by the senior students.

My education in the appropriate behavior of a student during my first year of study took many forms. For instance, one day, I asked Kanriye Fujima if we could spend some time in the afternoon after lessons to discuss her life in Japan. She agreed, but when I started asking questions about life in Japan following World War II, Barbara Uyesugi began vacuuming Kanriye's living room. The noise was so loud we could not hear each other. Kanriye Fujima, without indicating my question was inappropriate, concluded the interview by saying it was time for my lesson, even though I had already had a lesson that morning and was not scheduled to take another that afternoon. Each of us, including Kanriye, Barbara, and Miyoko, all went to our rooms to put on our practice attire. As Miyoko and I were waiting for Kanriye Fujima to come into the studio, Miyoko asked me if I knew anything about Japanese etiquette. She did not explain to me where I had erred, but asked in a tone of voice that indicated I was expected to discover the answer. I was left to think about it. Ultimately, I realized I had been pressing my inquiries into topical areas that were considered intrusive. This was confirmed for me later when Barbara Uyesugi revealed to me that in the Japanese training system a student never asks personal questions of her teacher. Although Barbara had worked with Kanriye Fujima for thirty years she had never discussed her teacher's personal life with her.

Besides teaching me the correct behavior they also constantly found ways of helping me to focus on the material which they deemed important for me to know. An incident occurred one afternoon while I was observing Kanriye Fujima teach a lesson. On the days she was teaching in Portland, I would arrive in the morning just prior to the first student's lesson and spend the entire day both watching other people's lessons and taking my own. On most days the three senior students--Barbara, Micki, and Miyoko--were also there. On one occasion when I had just finished taking a lesson, Kanriye Fujima indicated that I should be certain to write down the portion I had just learned so I would not forget it. I began to write down a portion of the dance, but became distracted because I was also trying to record my observations of the lesson currently taking place. Miyoko asked me if I was writing down my dance piece. I replied that I was writing down observations of the current student's lesson. Her only reply was "Oh!" spoken with such obvious disappointment that I knew that in some manner I had not fulfilled her expectations of me. It was only later after many such incidents that I realized my behavior was always rewarded when I consciously focused on learning and recording the dance pieces that Kanriye Fujima was teaching me.

Kanriye Fujima's quiet persistence left me with a choice. I could adopt her approach to the student-teacher relationship which would influence my approach as a researcher or I could continue to pursue a more clinical social science research posture. In attempting to decide how or if I should continue the study, I was influenced by recent critiques of the accepted relationship between ethnographer and informant.

Although most ethnographers have included discussions in their field notes of this interviewer-informant dialogue, it is only within the last twenty years that these discussions have been published. Current interest in this dialogue has been partly a response to ethnographic writing since the publication of Edward Said's book *Orientalism* in 1979. Two writers who have voiced specific criticisms of earlier ethnographic texts are Renato Rosaldo (1986) and George Marcus (1986). They consider past relationships between ethnographers and the people with whom they have been working to have been a continuation of the hegemonic nature of colonial relationships, which tend to view a specific group through the lens of their social groups' fantasies about that group. A fantasy often perpetuated by the popular culture. James Clifford argues that the problem with past ethnographic research and writing is the position of the ethnographer in relationship to the subject of research, the ethnographer taking on the role of omniscient observer, while the subject of research becomes the object of study. With the completion of the published ethnography it is the writer's voice which pervades, effectively distancing the subjects of research from their initial contribution. A second critique is aimed at the assumption on the part of most ethnographers that they can maintain a disinterested distance between themselves and the people with whom they are working. As George Marcus puts it:

> The figure of the primitive or the alien other is no longer as compelling as it was in similar experimental periods. Global homogenization is more credible than ever before, and though the challenge to discover and represent cultural diversity is strong, doing so in terms of spatio-temporal cultural preserves of otherness seems outmoded. (Marcus, 1986, p. 168)

Marcus and Rosaldo advocate an approach that is, from a theatrical standpoint, a "Brechtian" approach to ethnography. That is, the ethnographer as Brechtian actor constantly points out to the reader of his text the ethnographer's role in it. The value of this approach to ethnography is realized in the potential for increased dialogue between interviewer and informant. "Once cultures are no longer prefigured visually--as objects, theaters, texts--it becomes possible to think of a cultural poetics that is an interplay of voices, of positioned utterances" (Clifford, 1986, p. 12).

In the past ten years, partly as a response to these criticisms, several sociologists and anthropologists including Langness and Frank (1981), Crapazano (1980), Plummer (1983), and McAdams (1985) have discussed these problems extensively as related both to the development of life histories and case studies. They have considered the methods of solving the primary problems of accuracy in collecting data and the methods of analysis of that data, and have focused on such ideas as the role of the relationship between the researcher and the subject of the research (Crapazano, Langness and Frank); how one examines a total life through specific themes (Langness and Frank), or archetypes (McAdams); or simply how the researcher both establishes intimacy and maintains objectivity while using the data to direct the information towards a larger body of theory (Plummer).

Influenced by these contemporary critiques of the relationship between researcher and subject of research, I decided to reorient my approach to the fieldwork. Kanriye Fujima became not only a guide to my learning process of *nihon buyo* but also the director of the research. My role as a participant observer moved from being an observer who participates to a participant who observes. I concluded that it was only by becoming immersed within the training system as an active student-participant, within the perimeters created by Kanriye Fujima, would I understand her life's work and her impact on the students she teaches.

Analytic Approach

This book is my explication of Kanriye Fujima's teaching. It is an interpretation grounded in the experience of being a student. As mentioned, my field experience was a study very much directed by Kanriye Fujima. To the extent that she was in control of the amount and quality of information, it is her story as she wishes it to be told. Beyond participation as a student, the study is based on formal and informal interviews with other members of the school and a written performance record kept by Kanriye and the Portland based school Fujinami-kai. The analysis of her influence on her students is guided by my understanding founded upon experience as an instructor of theatre movement in the training of the psychophysical self.

Theatre movement training has evolved throughout the twentieth century as a system of training that defines the individualized self as a unification of mind and body. This specialty area of theatre has been guided by a group of movement theorists, many of whom are specialists in various aspects of the bodily disciplines, who consider people not as a mechanical set of individual parts but as a unified being. This trend is the reverse of the Cartesian approach to people which divides lived experience into two separate areas of knowing; one based on the rational mental processes of the brain and the other on information derived from the senses. This perspective assumes that there is a coherence in the interaction between the mind and the body. As Mark Johnson points out in *The Body in the Mind* (1987):

> Our reality is shaped by the patterns of our bodily movement, the contours of our spatial and temporal orientation, and the forms of our interaction with objects. It is never merely a matter of abstract conceptualizations and propositional judgments. (Johnson, 1987, p. xix)

Johnson explores the bodily basis of meaning, imagination, and reason by demonstrating the sensory base of many metaphors. He maintains that there is an initial physical base of metaphors such as 'balance of forces.' He suggests the concept of balance is physically based in our learning to discover our balance while learning to walk. Consequently according to Johnson, our understanding of our world and our ability to imagine other potential realties is influenced by the physical experiences we have had of it.

Michael Murphy's book *The Future of the Body* (1992)[5] documents this viewpoint in the work of theorists in the field of psychoanalytical and body therapy who have created a variety of approaches for solving psychological and physical problems through focusing on primarily physical approaches to therapy. The healing techniques, which rely on the sensory level of learning, knowledge, and understanding, are referred to as the somatic therapies.[6] They include the work of William Reich, Moshe Feldenkrais, F. M. Alexander, Ida Rolph, Edmund Jacobson, Charlotte Selver, and others. Although each technique focuses on a specific method, they regard the self as a cybernetic system in which all parts of the self are in a state of constant interaction. They operate on the premise that:

> Not only is it true that the nervous system stimulates the body to move in specific ways as a result of specific sensations; it is also the case that all movements flood the nervous system with sensations regarding the structures and functions of the body. Movement is the unifying bond between the mind and the body, sensations are the substance of the bond. (Juhan, 1987, p. xxv)

Whether active or passive in its method of working with the individual, the intent of each somatic technique is to retrain the psychophysical self. The individual and group experiences promote some or all of the following:

sensory and kinesthetic awareness; control of autonomic processes; efficient modulation of sensory input; sensorimotor coordination; the articulation and coordination of particular muscle groups; grace and efficiency of posture, carriage, and movement; new patterns of movement; flexibility of facial and gestural expression; general relaxation as well as the relaxation of particular body parts during complex behaviors; recuperation from stress; vitality; awareness and control of emotions and mental processes; sensory, kinesthetic, emotional, and intellectual pleasure. (Murphy, 1992, p. 414)

Proponents of Reichian derived psychoanalytic therapy contend that personality is manifested in the musculature of the body. Often referred to as bioenergetics, a portion of the therapy consists of a series of physical exercises, the purpose of which is to help to break down the musculature armoring of the client which will theoretically result in a change of personality.

The philosophic foundation of the somatic therapies is a western version of Asian epistemological approaches to the nature of knowledge. The western distrust of sensory information encouraged a system of learning and transference of information that privileged verbal rather than nonverbal forms of communication. Consequently students are taught all forms of material, including theatre, through methods that depend upon auditory and visual learning. Eastern training strategies incorporate kinesthetic methods of training as well as visual and auditory.

The result is a tradition of individual transmission of cultural information, including theatre, which relies not on a single learning modality such as aural, visual, or kinesthetic, but in a method of training that incorporates all three. Phillip Zarrilli refers to this form of teaching as 'in-body' learning:

> The process of transmission of performance knowledge in such disciplines is one of constant repetition where the neophyte literally mimics the master. Day after day the student repeats over and over again the techniques of the system under the watchful eye of the master. (Zarrilli, 1990, p. 133)

This method of teaching is not limited to pre-twentieth century Asian theatre forms, but is currently part of the training method used by modern Japanese theatre practitioner Tadaki Suzuki. James Brandon observes:

> The system is very Japanese. No one speaks a word except Suzuki. No one asks a question. No one makes a suggestion. The acknowledged star of the group, Kayoko Shiraishi, an actress of terrifying force on the stage, is indistinguishable among the other performers. There is an electric alertness, a quiet tension in the room. They accept shouted criticism, slaps on the head, calls of 'damned fool' (*baba yaro*). Suzuki is their teacher, their sensei. In this respect the Waseda Little Theatre is following attitudes toward learning a 'way' (*do*) and the strict master-pupil relationship that is typical of traditional arts of all kinds in Japan. (Brandon, 1987, p. 30-31)

Using verbal cues to indicate the appropriate rhythmic emphasis, the typical teacher of an Asian theatrical form situates him/herself in front of the students and repeats the movement phrases again and again while the students attempt to follow. This method of instruction encourages a high level of concentration as the students incorporate all their learning modalities in order to successfully follow the information the teacher is communicating by primarily nonverbal means. Over an extensive period of study the student's muscle memory becomes encoded with the movement associated with a theatrical style. The average Japanese student continues studying for a lifetime.

There is an assumption that the student will not only learn the form but will be transformed psychologically as well:

> A common assumption of these disciplines is that each is a psychophysical means to effecting a fundamental transformation in the individual: the martial arts effected an actual transformation from a raw, unknowledgeable, inexperienced, unconcentrated, unskilled youth to a seasoned, 'knowledgeable,' experienced, concentrated, integrated, skilled warrior capable of 'conquering even the god of death.' (Zarrilli, 1990, p. 132-133)

The students are transformed from one psychophysical state to another through a systematic method of training that in its constant imitation of the teacher causes them to incorporate their entire being into the process of learning.[7] This form of training I refer to as *somatic training* as it requires moment to moment interaction of the physical and neural systems through the aural, visual, and kinesthetic means of knowing. Borrowing from Zarrilli, I refer to the actual learning, as differentiated from the training method, as *embodied learning*.

The decision, to be directed by Kanriye Fujima in the organization of the research, necessitated that I apply my training in the somatic disciplines during the field experience. Instead of concentrating primarily on information I was given verbally through interviews, I needed to understand the information I was being given nonverbally through lessons. Therefore, part of the field research consisted of spending many hours practicing the dance theatre pieces she was teaching me. I tried, while repeating the pieces, to understand the reason Kanriye Fujima taught me any particular piece. What was there about my own personality and physical movement tendencies which caused her to teach me this specific dance rather than another one? I tried to monitor my emotional reaction to learning different kinds of dances and different kinds of dramatic characters associated with each dance. I also had to integrate the movement information with the verbal explanations of the dance pieces. Finally, I had the opportunity to extend my experience by performing in Portland and Ontario with other members of the school.

While living in Ontario, I realized that the training techniques (somatic and otherwise) which Kanriye Fujima applied to me are those she applies to all of her American students regardless of ethnic background. Like the movement style she teaches, they are very subtle, and often rely on a seeming lack of direction and revolve around several skills which are primary to the high-context[8] Japanese culture. Her unwillingness to speak English with her students is one of her primary methods of forcing students to develop concentration and attention to the nonverbal cues around them. Being taught a set of movement phrases (*kata*) through physical imitation rather than verbal descriptions helps students to develop a high level of somatic awareness. This increased level of awareness is an asset to them in absorbing large amounts of nonverbal cues within social situations as well as when learning dances. Kanriye Fujima's firm insistence on the customary behavior modes, including specific dress and deportment among all students according to their position within the school, reinforces a general acceptance of the individual's position within their social milieux. The dance pieces she selects for each student are intended to teach them a physical skill such as strength or dexterity, or a personal quality such as physical and verbal silence.

Informal conversations with other students helped me to realize how much we shared a common process. They were also Americans, who for the most part did not speak Japanese, did not know the history behind the pieces or many of the Japanese traditional art forms (flower arranging and calligraphy) portrayed in the dances. However there were also two clear differences. First, the majority of the students were exploring a past they had unconscious if not conscious knowledge about through their heritage as Japanese Americans. I, on the other hand, albeit with more formal knowledge of Japanese culture and of the interrelationship between mind and body, was not a member of their ethnic group. Secondly, even though I was committed to being a student, I was also an academic who had a tendency to focus more on asking the question than experiencing the moment. It was Kanriye Fujima's subtle insistence that the answers to the questions I was asking was not in a discussion of the form but in a pursuit of it that helped me to understand what I was observing and experiencing.

John Blacking in his introductory chapter to *Towards an Anthropology of the Body* (1977) remarks:

> The shared states of different bodies can generate different means of repeated movements in space and time that can be transmitted from one generation to another. Thus an infinite number of cultural variations are possible, based on the variables of shared somatic states, movements of the body, numbers and shapes of organisms involved, dimensions of space and durations of time. (Blacking, 1977, p.9)

This statement is a result of the research of numerous twentieth century anthropologists who have observed that cultural ideas are not only embedded in our psyche but have expression in our physical beings. Our postures, gestures, experiences of time, and space are all a result of our enculturation in a specific social group.

Participants in a social group learn the appropriate nonverbal interactional behaviors through daily participation in the society a part of which includes performance forms.[9] As a performance medium, Asian dance theatre is a complex set of symbolic information that involves various stages and levels of interaction from the training of performers to live performance. Each stage of the process engages the participants in the interchange and transmission of deeply held cultural values. Teachers accepted as authorities of the form and by extension 'transmitters of culture' train students in the psychological and physical components of the form. The public performance on a stage situated in a unique time and space becomes the symbolic enactment of the group's system of values.

This study is an examination of the methods used by Kanriye Fujima to teach the Japanese dance theatre form *nihon buyo* in the United States. Chapter two sets the scene by recounting her early life in Japan in relationship to the development of *nihon buyo* in the twentieth century. The third chapter delineates the basic movement style and its associated aesthetic ideals. The fourth chapter considers the students backgrounds who study the form. Chapter five describes the organization of the studio as well as the process of teaching. The sixth chapter explores the performance elements and their influence on the student's learning process. Chapter seven is a description of several contexts of performance in the three communities in which she has taught. The final chapter is a discussion of Kanriye Fujima's retention of specific components of the tradition in which she was trained, her impact on the students and the communities in which she works.

Notes

1. *Nihon buyo* is a twentieth-century theatrical form sometimes referred to as *kabuki buyo* which has its direct roots in the *kabuki* theatre of the sixteenth century as well as indirect roots in the *noh* theatre of the fifteenth century, and the *kagura* rituals of the seventh century.

2. Shoes are consistently removed when entering most Japanese homes. Prior to the twentieth century the removal of the shoes in Japan was a means of protecting the tatami mat grass floors. It is a custom that I have observed in many homes of Japanese Americans.

3. To call an individual sensei (teacher) in the systems of traditional Japanese training is to acknowledge a relationship of duty and trust between the student and teacher.

4. I continue to maintain my membership in Fujinami-kai and travel to Portland or Ontario whenever my responsibilities at the University of California permit it.

5. This is the most complete study of the variety of body-mind approaches that have gained recognition in the last thirty years. It includes discussions of the approaches and the related laboratory research.

6. The use of the term soma or somatic to refer to the integration of the mind and body was developed by philosopher Thomas Hanna and is discussed in *Bodies in Revolt: A Primer in Somatic Thinking* (New York: Holt, Rinehart, and Winston, 1970).

7. I would maintain that the modifications of the psychophysical nature of the individual beyond concentration and mind-body integration will depend upon the movement qualities associated with the theatrical form. For although there may be similarities in teaching style between Asian theatre disciplines, a student of one of the Indian Sanskrit drama forms is not learning through a similar training style the same aesthetic information as expressed in its cultural-physical complex as a student of Japanese theatre.

8. High context is a term coined by Edward Hall to refer to groups of people who rely heavily on nonverbal elements in conversation. The European American population of the United States is by contrast a low context culture. Edward Hall, *The Hidden Dimension* (New York: Anchor Books, 1969).

9. A discussion of the application of proxemics to theatre from a semiotic standpoint can be found in Hodge, R. and Kress, G., *Social Semiotics* (Cambridge: Polity Press, 1988).

CHAPTER II

KANRIYE FUJIMA'S LIFE

AND

TRADITIONAL JAPANESE DANCE THEATRE

Smiling from the front pages of the arts section of a western Oregon newspaper one October morning in 1987 was the face of traditional Japanese theatre performer Kanriye Fujima. It was not the first time the story of her life and teaching had appeared in a Pacific Northwest newspaper, for she had been the subject of many articles in Portland, Oregon; Spokane, Washington; and in her adopted community of Ontario, Oregon. Each time one of the three communities in which she has taught sponsors a recital, or one of the *buyo* schools performs at a community-sponsored international festival or at a local Japanese community festival, the local press has referred to the life and work of Kanriye Fujima. But the article mentioned above was the first time the public press had acknowledged the thirty plus years she had devoted to teaching in Oregon and Washington.

Kanriye Fujima's life is a story of a woman who says "My life is dance and I love my life." It is also a story of the women who have worked with her over the years and have gone to Japan to become *natori*. Finally, it is the story of three generations of students who have studied *nihon buyo* with the woman they all call 'Sensei.'

Early Years in Yamaguchi

Like many people raised in Japan, Kanriye Fujima is hesitant to talk about the details of her life. However, during many afternoon tea breaks and two formal interviews, she shared with me the general profile of her life as it pertains to her career as a student and teacher of *nihon buyo*. It is a complex narrative which includes the story of her life, the history of artistic tradition in which she was trained, and the changing relationship between Japan and the United States.

Kanriye Fujima was born in 1923 during the reign of Emperor Taisho or the Taisho period in Yamaguchi, a Japanese province located near Hiroshima in the southern portion of the main island of Honshu. When she was very young or as she puts it a "100 days old" her father died, and some time after that her mother remarried. In 1929 at the auspicious age of six, during the strategic sixth month of June, she began studying classical Japanese dance/theatre with the Yamamura school.[1] A short time later she began studying singing and *shamisen*, the instrument which is the major accompaniment for most of the classical Japanese dance/theatre pieces. The Yamamura school in which she studied was one of the old schools of classic dance or *odori*. It was founded by Tomogoro (1718-1844) in the first half of the nineteenth century. With its main headquarters in the Kansai region or Kyoto-Osaka area, it was a school active during the Meiji period not only in the *kabuki* theatre world but due to the efforts of the second Tomogoro and the two adopted daughters of the first Tomogoro "in the geisha quarters and among the townsmen" (Kasho, 1969, p. 352).

When Kanriye Fujima began her study of *buyo*, the form *nihon buyo* was in the process of solidifying itself after the years of innovation initiated by the Meiji Restoration in 1868 and the intense westernization that this political change stimulated. At the beginning of the Meiji period dance existed in numerous areas of Japanese life. There were the religious *kagura* performances at shinto shrines, the ritualized *bugaku* performances at court, the dance portions of *noh* and *kabuki* theatre, and the folk dances associated with yearly festivals such as *obon*. The primary ferment was not in the religious, court or folk performances or even in the *noh* theatre but in the popular *kabuki* theatre out of which would evolve *nihon buyo*.

Kabuki, the popular theatre of the middle class, was considered until the Meiji period a second class citizen in comparison to the *noh* theatre of the aristocracy.[2] But the status of *kabuki* changed dramatically in 1887 when the Emperor indicated his acceptance of the form by attending a performance. *Kabuki* immediately became a "classical theatre." *Kabuki* actors, who until then had been considered 'river bed beggars,' became, overnight, purveyors of a classical form.

Kabuki, a four hundred year old form, was originally developed in the early 1600s by Okuni, a priestess of the Izumo shrine. In response to the dictates of the popular culture and the will of the shogunate during any given period, *kabuki* had developed by the Meiji Restoration into a complex form which included spoken drama, an interweaving of spoken drama and dance, and dramatic dance pieces referred to as *shosagoto*. The actors for both male and female characters were the male members of families who in the highly stratified Japanese theatre society specialized in acting. The female equivalent of the male *kabuki* actor were the *o-kyogenshi* who taught and sometimes presented plays in the women's quarters of noble houses. However, during the Meiji Restoration these women teacher/performers lost their noble following. "Some of them became actresses and played in the provinces, some moved from job to job, some went to ruin" (Kasho, 1969, p. 357).

The dance element of *kabuki* was overseen by actor/choreographers or *furitsukeshi*. This was a result of the increasing complexity of *kabuki* as a theatre form in the seventeenth century. The history of *kabuki* choreographers has been an intricate interweaving of the ascendancy of one family followed by another. Various families dominated the field of choreography during the Tokugawa period (1603-1868), but by the Meiji Restoration the most noted were Jusuke Hanayagi founder of the Hanayagi school and Kan'emon Fujima II. Jusuke Hanayagi was the son of an Edo toy merchant who was fond of theatre. Jusuke started taking dancing lessons from *kabuki* actor Senzo Nishikawa. As an adult Jusuke developed a professional relationship with the powerful Danjuro family which led to his appointment as the permanent dance master on the staff of the Ichimura-za theatre in Edo. He founded during this period his own school of dance and *kabuki* choreography which continues to be one of the primary exponents of the form. Kan'emon Fujima II was the continuation of the line founded by Kambei. Kambei was a seventeenth century *no kyogen* actor, who came from a village called Fujima. (Kincaid, 1925) He became one of the early *kabuki* choreographers and the family has continued their prominence in the field through the twentieth century. Other schools in existence, but which did not dominate, were the Nishikawa school in Nagoya, the Katayama (later known as Inoe), Umemoto and Yamamura schools of Kansai area.

The primacy of these schools as the major exponents of dance was particularly challenged during the Meiji period by two people. One of these people was dramatist-critic Shoyo Tsubouchi (1859-1935). In 1894 he decided to revolutionize the traditional style of dance associated with *kabuki*. He invited Chuji Nishikawa, a *o-kyogenshi* and an actress, who performed with a troupe at the home of a *daimyo* (lord), to teach his children. On observing the style of movement she taught, he decided to create a new dance-drama style based on the movement style of *kabuki*. In 1904 he published *New Music Drama Theory* based on his knowledge of *kabuki* dance and western opera. Unfortunately, his original choreography, *Shinkyoku urashima* (New Urashima), was not well received. He returned in 1908 to a more traditional style *kabuki* movement in the creation of his later works, the most famous of which is *Onatsu kyoran* (The Madness of Onatsu) based on the seventeenth century love story of Onatsu and Seijuro. (Gunji, 1970)

During this same period, Shizue Fujima or Shizuki Fujikage, as she was later called, decided to become a professional dancer after seeing a performance of *Musume dojo-ji* by Ichikawa Kumehachi. At the age of 19 in 1899, she became Kumehachi's student, and later the student of Kan'emon Fujima. The all-male world of professional *kabuki* actors refused to accept her, so she joined the 'floating world' of professional entertainers called *geisha*.[3] In 1917, after she had completed paying her contractual debt to her employer at the tea house where she worked, Shizue, with the assistance of Kanji Fujima, a student colleague, organized a dance company called Fujikage-kai so she could create new dance pieces based on traditional theatre movement. In 1921, one of her pieces entitled *Shinbon* (Everyday Thoughts), "caused such a sensation among the critics that even the foremost *kabuki* actors of the day took notice of it and attended Shizue's performances" (Gunji, 1970, p. 177).

The popularity of her performance pieces influenced the *kabuki* actors to begin to give dance performances separate from *kabuki* programs; however, these performances were not as well received as those of Shizue Fujima. Shizue, with the continued support of her teacher Kan'emon, created a number of new dances based on *kabuki* movement. Ultimately, it was Shizue and other women who became the founders of the new dance movement, *nihon buyo*. *Kabuki* actor choreographer, Jusuke Hanayagi II, incorporated these women into the traditional *kabuki* world by giving them permission to become choreographers. His decision was intensely opposed by the conservative *kabuki* families who insisted that *kabuki* had always been the province of men. The women who had passed the Hanayagi exam were during this period not allowed to perform under the schools name.[4] However, other *kabuki* actors and actor/choreographers such as Koisaburo Hishikawa, Kanjuro Fujima, Juraku Hanayagi, and Tokubei Hanayagi, broke with tradition and became active in *nihon buyo* as they realized that training women as dancers was a means of extending their influence beyond the typical *kabuki* audience. They established schools of *nihon buyo* with themselves as the headmasters.

During this period women could be trained within the schools associated with *kabuki* but they could never become headmasters in any of the established schools. The headmaster position was limited to the direct male descendant of the current male headmaster. Schools in which there were only female heirs as next of kin when the head of the school died adopted someone from another school to replace the previous headmaster. An example of this is the Fujima school:

> The Fujima school, being without a male successor for a period, lost its place to the Nishikawa and Hanayagi schools. A pupil of the Fujima school, one Fujima Kan'emon, restored it to prominence at the end of the Tokugawa era, being encouraged by Ichikawa Danjuro IX, to become a Kabuki choreographer, and the school has retained an important position in the Kabuki world ever since. (Scott, 1955, p. 85-86)

During the Meiji period there were also schools of dance that were not associated with *kabuki*. One example is the Inoue School of Kyoto founded by Yachiyo Inoue I. She had taught *mai*, a dance style derived from *noh*, to members of the aristocratic Konoe family and to ladies-in-waiting at the imperial court. Influenced by conflicts within the traditional theatre, she also established her own Inoue school with herself as head. Following her and Shizue Fujima's example, other women have during the course of the twentieth century separated themselves from their original teachers and formed their own schools. Their primary motivation in doing so was the desire to realize their own work. All of the schools, regardless of origin, operate under the headmaster/student or *iemoto* system used for all traditional artistic forms in Japan. In Japan today there are more than 300 separate schools functioning under the broad umbrella of *nihon buyo*, some are extensions of schools associated with prominent *kabuki* actor-choreographers, others have developed out of court and folk forms of movement, and still others are offshoots of the first two. The schools associated with *kabuki* such as the Fujima or Hanayagi schools are headed by men. Other schools such as Inoue School of Kyoto are headed by women. Further recognition of *nihon buyo* as a form related to but separate from *kabuki* came in 1931 with the founding of the Japanese Dance Association.

The increased number of schools of dance in the 1920s coincided with Kanriye Fujima's study of *buyo*. It also coincided with the development of a middle-class who could afford to have their daughters study one of the classical art forms. The parents' goal was to prepare their daughters through the study of the arts for their responsibilities as adults. They also believed education in the arts would help them to find more attractive marriage partners. Therefore young women were encouraged by their families to study what was at that time called *odori*, along with flower arranging, classical music, and the tea ceremony. As a student, the daughter would develop qualities such as *seishin* or spiritual strength through the study of an artistic discipline that would help her to cope with "the demands and realities of everyday life" (Hendry, 1987, p. 158). She would also gain an ability to concentrate on a task and to demonstrate skill in a specific area.

Each afternoon Kanriye Fujima left the public school to enter the world of Japanese dance theatre. The individual discipline required as part of this consistent regimen was not always easy for a young girl of six to follow. One hot summer day as she started on her way to her *shamisen* lesson, she decided to take a vacation from daily practice and to go swimming instead. Unfortunately, she left her *shamisen* on top of the roof, and when she returned, the fragile instrument had been irreparably damaged. The response of her parents, especially her step-father, was predictable. She was reprimanded and told to concentrate on her lessons. As children do, she resisted his instructions but was glad as an adult that he "pushed me to practice both *odori* and *shamisen*." Kanriye Fujima continued to study through her teen-age years; however, from the beginning her talent for dance exceeded her ability as a singer/musician, and with the death of her first teacher when she was 15, she decided to concentrate primarily on *buyo*.

Student and Teacher in Japan

In the middle of this period in 1938 after the death of her first teacher, Kanriye Fujima went to live as an *uchi deshi* (live in student) in the home of her new teacher from the Yamamura school. Kanriye Fujima's responsibilities as a *deshi*, beyond being a student, involved care of various portions of the household and all aspects of the care of her teacher's children, including the unpleasant job of changing the babies' diapers. She was also responsible for helping the teacher instruct some of her students who came to her home, as well as teaching for groups like the Japanese Railway Employees Union. She stayed with this teacher for three years but decided to leave in 1941 as "the teacher wanted to control all aspects of my life and I did not want that."

The system Kanriye entered by assuming the role of *uchi deshi* was codified during the Tokugawa period, by families associated with the arts. It was, and is, a set of relationships currently referred to as the *iemoto* system. The *iemoto* system, structured like a Japanese family, became the vehicle for the transmission of the artistic 'skill' from one generation to another. Francis Hsu identifies it as a kin-tract system:

> By this term I refer to a fixed and unalterable hierarchial arrangement voluntarily entered into among a group of human beings who follow a common code of behavior under a common ideology for a set of common objectives. (Hsu, 1975, p. 62)

The system had four primary structural features; 1) a master-student relationship, 2) an interlinking hierarchy, 3) the supreme authority of the *iemoto*, and, 4) the *iemoto* as a pseudo-family system. One author describes it in relationship to *joruri* singers:

> It is not merely an organization, but offers a way of life, a framework for structuring that life, and a strategy for dealing with internal dissension and external pressures. The *iemoto* is a hierarchial system in which one person, in this case Ayanosuke acts as the focus of loyalty from ranked disciples and other followers. These individuals such as students, audience members, relatives, patrons and fellow artists form a group similar to a family and play a significant role in the survival of the *iemoto*. (Coaldrake, 1989, p. 159)

Albeit the system when Kanriye Fujima joined it as a student was a part of male dominated public theatre, similar organizational structures had existed both in female performance groups associated with the Shinto temples and in the family structure prior to the Tokugawa period. For example, there were groups of women priestesses in pre-Buddhist Japan (prior to AD 700) who were associated with the Shinto temples and performed *kagura* rituals to make the gods happy. They lived in *miko-mura* or *miko* villages near the shrines. "From these bases they would set out at stated seasons of the year on long peripatetic journeys, like strolling minstrels, delivering prophesies and messages from the dead in the villages they passed" (Blacker, 1975, p. 127). At religious festivals the priestesses referred to as *miko* would start a dance which would give way to a trance in which she could communicate with the *kami* (gods). This early form of performance associated with the *miko* can be found occasionally today, but only on the seven Izu islands located west of Tokyo.

Later, in the Heian period (794-1185) the *asobi*, women members of a religious order, performed with a dual function of priestess and entertainer. They were singers of *imayo*, a form of folk song with a large repertoire taken from Buddhist mythology and peasant festival songs. They lived in and near shrines and were often sought out by court nobles, both in their capacity as singers and for their sexual favors. The *asobi* were organized similarly to the current *iemoto* system:

> As a group, *Asobi* seemed to have maintained a loose internal structure headed by a female leader at the top. These head mistresses are believed to have reached such positions by virtue of their superiority in their imayo skill and their personal charm as courtesans. It is not known exactly what functions these leaders had, but presumably these women were charged to protect their group members from undue exploitation by customers, to maintain certain order within the group, and sometimes to supervise the distribution of goods among themselves. (Kwon, 1988, p. 210)

Similar performance oriented groups of women, the *geisha* were formed in the late eighteenth century. (Dalby, 1983)

The *furitsukeshi* or *kabuki* choreographers, who had become identified as a special group in the eighteenth century, began in the nineteenth century to apply the *iemoto* model to their training of students. Scott describes the training in these early schools:

> Training was severe and a high level of accomplishment was not easily obtained. Many schools came into being and the successors of some of them still carry on the names today. The various schools gained their

theatrical supremacy through their popularity with the leading actor and the personalities of the chief choreographers, rather than through any marked differences in idea. Fundamentally they were all related, disciples of one school for instance might, and did, become the *iemoto* of a rival school. (Scott, 1955, p. 85)

The *iemoto* system operates like an extended family with members of a school calling themselves *uchi no mono*, or members of the same household. Teachers often refer to their students as their children. Hence, a highly personal relationship evolves between student and teacher based on a system of *on* (reciprocal obligations). The teacher is responsible for providing a model for the traditional form, acting as a transmitter of the philosophical and cultural aspects of the form, and providing educational experiences for the learner's self-discovery. The student's responsibility is to exhibit *nyunanshin* (pliant-heartedness) and apply herself as a student with diligence, respect, and perseverance. The attitude of the student toward the teacher and the form is *kansha* (gratefulness). "The sensei, who is in an emic position, accepts the student, who is in an etic position, because of the latter's desire to learn the art and progress along the path of spiritual education following traditional methods" (Schmidt, 1986, p. 73).

The system follows pyramidal structure with the *iemoto*/headmaster at the top of the pyramid. For instance, within the Fujima school of *nihon buyo*, the current *iemoto* is Kan'emon Fujima, one in a long line of *kabuki* actor-choreographers going back to the seventeenth century. Generally, teachers within the school are positioned in the hierarchy depending upon their relationship to the *iemoto*. Among family members the line is traced from oldest to youngest through males. Students who are not family members are placed in the hierarchy depending upon how close their relationship is to the *iemoto*.

The student of a traditional form is at first an apprentice who tacitly agrees to give control to his teacher of his/her education in the form. It is not expected that the student will question either the material taught or the method of teaching. The goal of the student is simply to duplicate the form as taught by the teacher. The position of the student is slightly changed when he or she passes a specific level of ability and moves from being considered an apprentice to an accomplished performer of the art form. In the world of *nihon buyo*, this transition takes place when the student performs a *fuji* (girl) and *matsu* (boy) piece before the *iemoto* and his/her representatives. Once they pass this exam, they are considered *natori* and are qualified to teach and perform under the school's name.

Because there is an assumption of blood relationship between members of the school the performance name they assume combines the name of the school with that of the teacher. For example, "in the Hanayagi School of dancing 'Hanayagi Sumi' would be the direct disciple of Hanayagi Suho, while 'Hanayagi Rokumi' is the direct disciple of Hanayagi Rokuji" (Hsu, 1975, p. 63). The use of the Hanayagi name indicates a direct relationship to that school and the similarity of the first syllable indicating the direct relationship to a specific teacher.

While living and training within this environment established by the *iemoto* system, Kanriye Fujima had learned a set of behaviors from working within this codified system of oral learning. Following a strict code of etiquette the student, on arrival at the teacher's house for a lesson, changed into her practice attire, consisting of *tabi* (sock like coverings for the feet), practice *kimono*, and *obi*. Once dressed, she sat at the side of the room in *seiza* and waited for a fellow student to finish her lesson. The student was expected to demonstrate respect, humility, and dedication by sitting quietly in *seiza* during any periods the teacher was not directly working with her. One demonstration of that respect was sitting at all times facing towards the teacher so that her feet never faced the teacher. When the teacher indicated she was ready for her, the student came to the center of the floor, sat in *seiza*, then knelt and bowed, saying *onegai shimasu*. The teacher indicated to her she was ready to begin, and the student stood to imitate the phrases taught by the teacher. At the end of the lesson, the student knelt and bowed again, saying *domo aragato gozaimashita* (thank you very much).

Before and After World War II

The period leading up to and following World War II was a difficult time for everyone in Japan. Pressures were placed on all forms of art by the military government during the 1930s and 40s to perform programs that validated the political position of the military. Performers, including Kanriye Fujima, became part of the government's military propaganda, being required to perform patriotic pieces for government-organized assemblies. The military demands also created shortages of all forms of consumer goods, including food. Even in the countryside where Kanriye Fujima lived, there was general hunger. The end of the war in 1946 did not automatically end the deprivations associated with it. The country and its populace had to come to terms with the consequences of the war which included both continued limited resources and adapting to the forces of the allied occupation.

During the early phase of the occupation Kanriye Fujima left Yamaguchi and went to live in the areas of Hiroshima that were being rebuilt following the atomic bomb blast of 1945. She had come to the conclusion that she wanted to become a professional *nihon buyo* teacher and believed that she needed further training in a school which was connected with *kabuki*. Thus, she went to Hiroshima to study with Kansho Fujima, a teacher from the highly regarded Fujima school.

With this move, Kanriye Fujima began a concentrated period of study in one of the foremost schools. The head of the Fujima school was *kabuki* actor Shoroku Onoe (his name as *iemoto* of the Fujima school was Kan'emon Fujima), one of the finest performers of *kabuki* then active. In 1949 Kanriye Fujima performed the two requisite dance pieces for Kan'emon in Tokyo and became licensed to teach in the Fujima school. The license also permitted her to take the name of the school, Fujima, as part of her own name. The transition from the Yamamura school to the Fujima school had been very difficult, for the Fujima movement style was more complex, but ultimately Kanriye Fujima believed it had been worth the work as she states "It allowed me more freedom."

After she became a licensed teacher, Kanriye taught in the Hiroshima area for seven years in a private studio in her home, taking on more aspects of the teaching than would have been normal in pre-war Japan. Prior to the war, the dance community was divided among separate families, with each family responsible for a different aspect of a *nihon buyo* production. There were different people who took care of make-up, costumes, music, and choreography. This system broke down during and after the war, as many of the people who had been responsible for specific aspects of the production were no longer available. In order for a program to be successful, Kanriye Fujima had to assume responsibility for these areas of production and in the process discovered that she enjoyed overseeing all aspects of performance. As she said in one interview, "I wanted to do all the things that went with the dance. I wanted to do the weaving and the kimonos and the make-up" (Thiele, 1987, p. 46). As Japan began to recover economically, there was a trend to rebuild the artistic stratification that existed prior to the war. Kanriye found this trend increasingly frustrating as it did not allow her to be involved with the total dance production to the degree she wished.

Immigration to the United States

In 1956 Hisako Kanai, a former student of Kanriye Fujima's who had married and moved to Portland, Oregon, returned to Hiroshima to visit, bringing with her Portland hotel owner Etaro Takaki. She introduced Etaro Takaki to Kanriye Fujima. The two discovered they enjoyed each other's company and were married in Japan the same year. Following the wedding, Kanriye Fujima made her first trip outside of Japan to her new home of Portland, Oregon, with a promise from her new husband that he would support her desire to teach *nihon buyo* in America. Unlike many people who might have been nervous about moving to a new country whose language they did not speak, Kanriye was excited about the opportunity to be exposed to a new environment. She believed she would have the freedom to be responsible for all aspects of the performance of *nihon buyo*, from teaching to making all artistic decisions related to performance.

Kanriye Fujima's introduction to life in the United States was unique in comparison to other female Japanese immigrants of the same time period. (Glenn, 1986; Nakano, 1990) She came to the United States not only as a wife but with the goal of teaching her art form in this country. Although faced with the same initial culture shock of adapting to a new environment, she was able to immediately immerse herself in establishing classes and preparing for the students' first public presentation.

On her arrival in Portland, Kanriye Fujima began teaching in one of the large ballrooms of the hotel owned by her husband in northwest Portland. Many of her original students were, like herself, Japanese women who had married Japanese American men. Some of the younger members were new or *Shin Issei* who had only been in the United States a short time. However, there were a few older *Issei* students. There was unspoken mutual empathy among this group of women who had all survived the war and its aftermath on both sides of the Pacific. Kanriye Fujima's initial students also included some *Nisei* children of the *Shin Issei* as well as older *Nisei* and their children who would rush to lessons after work and school.

As news of her teaching spread through the communities in the Pacific Northwest, Kanriye Fujima was asked to travel once a month to Ontario, Oregon to teach. Unfortunately her teaching stopped abruptly when her husband, Etaro, became ill with cancer and died in 1958. After his death Kanriye returned to Japan for the next eight months to reconsider her life. As part of the process, she took the second level of accreditation from the Fujima School. She decided that with or without a husband, her life's work would be to teach in the United States the art forms associated with *nihon buyo*. Prior to leaving Japan for the second time, she met with the *iemoto* of the school, Kan'emon Fujima, in Tokyo. His response to her decision was typical of a master of an art form in a culture highly imbued with zen philosophy. He advised her that although she would no longer be able to study consistently in Japan, an artist could learn from many things and "America would now be her teacher." She returned to the United States and began her life as a traveling teacher, dividing her life primarily between Portland and Ontario.

The Traveling Teacher from Ontario

The community of Ontario, Oregon, gained a new kind of status in 1960 with Kanriye Fujima's arrival. She came as a result of her marriage to local restaurant owner Minoru Fujita, who she met during one of her many teaching trips to Ontario. Kanriye Fujima's face breaks out in a wistful smile when she talks about her late second husband. She laughs as she relates the concern of others over a marriage to a man who was thirty-seven years older than she was. "A lot of people thought we would have problems because there was such a difference in our ages but he was very supportive of my teaching, and that was very important to me." And until his death in 1985 he was one of the major advocates of her life as a traveling teacher. He introduced her to members of the Spokane community, and she added this city to her monthly round of teaching.[5] Nevertheless, he rarely traveled with her, but instead remained in Ontario. Even though she had taught dance in Hiroshima, Japan, and Portland, Oregon, the move to Ontario in 1958 initiated an important segment of her life in which she would dedicate herself to years of teaching students in three different communities.

Shortly after she moved to Ontario her life assumed a seasonal pattern dictated by the weather. Beginning in March and continuing until the first snow falls (usually in November), Kanriye Fujima has traveled to each of the three communities, teaching one week each in Portland and Spokane then returning to Ontario for two weeks. The winters she spends in Ontario, teaching lessons in her home studio. Each February Kanriye Fujima returns to Japan to visit her mother, who lives in a traditional Japanese house next to her brother's home in Hiroshima.[6] While there, she uses the opportunity to learn newly created dances from Kansho Fujima, the woman who was her first teacher in the Fujima school, and from her daughter. When possible, she makes arrangements to perform at recitals

Chronology of Events

1868	Meiji period begins.
1912/ 1926	Buyo as a form separate from Kabuki develops due to performances of Fujima Shizue encouraged by playwright Tsubouchi Shoyo (1859-1935) who created the term Buyo from the Chinese characters for mai and odori.
1923	Kanriye Fujima born in the Yamaguchi Prefecture in Japan.
1925	Geisha of Tokyo began performing on stage separate from tea houses.
1929	Kanriye Fujima begins studying shamisen and odori.
1934	Kanriye Fujima studies in the Yamamura school living with her teacher.
1941/ 1946	World War II
1948	Kanriye Fujima moves to Hiroshima to study odori with member of the Fujima school. She becomes a natori in 1949.
1956	Kanriye Fujima first comes to United States.
1957	Kanriye Fujima returns to Japan for eight months and then returns to the United States after receiving a secondary teaching certificate from Fujima school.
1960	Kanriye Fujima marries Minoru Fujita and moves to Ontario, Oregon adding Spokane to her teaching schedule.
1983	Three students of Kanriye Fujima, Hisako Kanai, Barbara Uyesugi and Miyoko Stroup go to Japan and pass the first level exam to become natori.
1985	Minoru Fujita, Kanriye Fujima's husband dies.
1987	A thirtieth recital is held in Portland celebrating Kanriye Fujima's years of teaching in that community.
1991	Grand Kabuki comes to Portland Oregon. Recital in Portland by Fujinami-kai.

given by the school associated with Kansho Fujima in Hiroshima. Once she returns to United States in the spring, she resumes her life as a traveling teacher. When asked if she will ever return to live permanently in Japan, she replies, "No, that America is my home now. The many students I have taught in this country have become my extended family."

Kanriye Fujima's life is dance. There are very few days in which she is not involved in dance, either teaching, preparing for a recital, playing the *shamisen*, watching videotapes of performances of her students or performers from Japan, making the practice *kimono* worn by the dancers, or choreographing or staging a dance piece. The days can sometimes be very long, such as during final preparations for a recital or a special festival like *Obon*.

In Ontario, she lives in a split-level home that was a Christmas present from her second husband. It is located in a quiet residential area across from the high school and includes a large basement in which she has built a studio to teach lessons. Although much smaller than any western dance studio, the studio has the typical accouterments of other dance studios in the United States: a wooden floor, full-length mirrors covering two separate walls, and a tape recorder. But it also has a number of things not found in a western dance studio: a rack covered with practice *kasa* (parasols) and fans for student use; a stack of long wooden spears in the corner used to practice male dance pieces; a monitor and video player; and numerous pictures of her students and teachers in Japan and America. Her studio typifies her home in general--a blend of influences. The basic architecture is suburban American tract housing but the windows are covered on the inside with sliding rice paper panels and the walls have Japanese hangings and collections of Japanese art. Outside the front door a carefully shaped pine is the center piece of a rock garden. However, the furniture, carpeting, and appliances in the rest of the house are the same as in many American households.

Regardless of community Kanriye spends most of her days teaching. The morning session, from 9:00 to 12:00, generally consists of young children, primarily girls (she has very few male students) who come each day for the week that she is in their community. They are brought by their mothers, who sit on the far end of the basement studio and watch while the children take their lessons. About noon, she takes a break for lunch and returns to teaching at 1:00 or 1:30. In the afternoon she often schedules the *shamisen* lessons she also teaches.

The afternoon students include women who have flexible work schedules or are retired. The lessons are often broken up by a short break from teaching about 4:00 PM, when she has tea. During this time she and the other *natori*, if she is in Portland, sit drinking tea and discussing their lives in general and their lives in art. At 5:00 PM, those women who cannot come earlier begin to arrive. This group sometimes includes teen-agers. The typical teaching day ends between 7:30 and 9:00 PM, after which she eats a late dinner and watches video tapes from Japan. At the end of the week, she packs up her tapes, gets into her large roomy Plymouth Voyager, and goes to the next community, listening and singing along to tapes of popular Japanese songs on her car stereo as she drives across the flat expanses of eastern Oregon and Washington.

Kanriye Fujima's evenings during the winter months are spent at home in Ontario watching videotapes from Japan, ranging from classical theatre performances to Japanese soap operas. Often she will combine an evening of television with putting together a *kimono*, most of which is sewn by hand. Friday evenings are poker nights when a group of male and female friends gather in the snug environment of one of the group's living room to play penny-ante poker while the wind blows the snow around outside. During those days, when the harsh eastern Oregon winter will permit it, she enjoys shopping and often drives the sixty miles to Boise, Idaho. She has an eye for style and buys wardrobe combinations that are much more typical of a sophisticated metropolitan area than the small farming community of Ontario. Usually at least once during the winter, Miyoko Stroup or Barbara Uyesugi, senior students from Portland, will take a bus from Portland to spend a week or two studying with Kanriye Fujima in Ontario. While they are in Ontario she gives them daily lessons in *buyo* and *shamisen*.

When she is in Ontario, Kanriye Fujima is active in the local community life, which centers around a variety of different churches from Buddhist to Mormon. Most of the Japanese Americans belong either to the Buddhist Temple or the United Methodist church, and Kanriye Fujima helps prepare programs for both. Her students regularly perform at *matsuri*, festivals associated with the Buddhist temple. She has also used Japanese *buyo* movement to choreograph Christmas carols for the United Methodist Church's Christmas program.

The holiday period from Thanksgiving to New Year is celebrated with a series of dinners at the homes of close friends. However, on New Year's Day, *Oshogatsu*, it is customary for members of Kanriye Fujima's inner circle to gather at her home. This group consists of Kanriye Fujima's older students and their families as well as the local Buddhist minister. In 1990 I was invited to participate in this celebration.

The day was typical Ontario cold with the weather well below freezing. Kanriye's house was the opposite of the external environment as the wood stove pumped out heat which blended with the smells coming from the kitchen. The living room was decorated for the occasion with customary Japanese New Year's decorations including the small *kadomatsu* shrine (an arrangement of pine and bamboo to ward off evil and evoke blessings) on top of the television with a drawing of herons for good luck. The *shimenawa*, the sacred rope of the sun-goddess Amaterasu, was draped over doors and areas of the living room. As each quest arrived they exchanged their street shoes for one of the many set of slippers waiting by the door.

A congenial atmosphere prevailed as each additional arrival remarked on the pleasure at being in the warmth of the home and out of the bitter January cold. Just prior to eating, Kanriye Fujima gathered everyone together and each person was offered a little *sake* out of the wide flat porcelain cups reserved especially for the New Year's celebration. The men were served first and all the other guests according to age. After the sake was served, the champagne was opened and glasses were poured for everyone. We all wished each other a good New Year in a mixture of Japanese and English while each took turns taking group pictures to record the event.

The large dining room table was covered with a large variety of foods, the most important of which was the fresh sea food which had been flown in from Japan and cut in a variety of styles to be served raw. There were several forms of *osechi ryori* (New Year's holiday food) besides the raw fish including *daikon* (radish), pickled vegetables, *mochi-gashi* (sweet pounded rice cakes) and bowls full of white rice. Everyone helped themselves and with plates appropriately filled found a seat in the attached living room. The room filled with the buzz of several quiet conversations concerning the success of the past year and the welfare of individual family members.

As each person finished eating they brought their china plates into the kitchen where a crew of volunteers was quickly cleaning up. All those not engaged in cleaning settled to watch a video tape version of the Japanese "Star Search" with a variety of singers from rock and roll to ballad. The dining table cleared, everyone found a chair and gathered around the table as the group settled down to concentrate on penny-ante poker. The rest of the day into the late evening hours disappeared in a series of raised bets as the Japanese singers continued to perform via video tape.

The time Kanriye Fujima does not spend either on the road teaching or living in Ontario is spent visiting family in Japan or Los Angeles. Although she and her husband had no children, his son by a former marriage has become like a son to her. She visits his family in Los Angeles regularly, attending important family gatherings such as her granddaughter Minna's graduation from the University of California at Los Angeles. These family visits are mutual, with visits by her stepson to Ontario and the family's attendance at her important recitals, including the one in which Kanriye Fujima performed in Hiroshima, Japan, in the fall of 1988.

Choices and Accommodations

Born in Japan at the beginning of the Taisho Period, Kanriye Fujima was a student of *nihon buyo* during the period of its development as an extension of the all male *kabuki* world. She lived through the tumultuous war years and the occupation that followed. She emigrated to the United States with a specific goal to teach *nihon buyo*. The life she has constructed in the United States blends the Japan of her youth with the influences of contemporary America. This blend is reflected in the diversity of the style of her split-level home.

Her move to the United States allowed her to continue the tradition of the form in which she was trained, but in an individual manner. Life in the United States allows her to be involved in every step, from teaching to costume repair. The new country also contained an established Japanese American community that was eager for the opportunity to come to understand through the study of traditional theatre the Japanese portion of their Japanese American background. The geographic barrier of the Pacific Ocean allowed her to explore areas of the art which would not have been possible in Japan.

The move to the Pacific Northwest allowed Kanriye Fujima to build her own world without severing her connection to the traditional schools in Japan. She brought from her Japanese heritage an extensive experience in the world of traditional Japanese dance theatre. This encompassed a method of organizing the relationship between teacher and students; the dances and movement style of the Yamamura and Fujima schools; the process of transmitting this information to a new group of students; and, a belief in the importance of the artistic training for the developing personality of her students. Influenced by both societies, she has maintained her membership within the Fujima school of Japan, yet developed schools in the Pacific Northwest.

Notes

1. The number six is an important part of the Japanese cultural belief system.

A child who starts studying a form at six within the sixth month is bound to succeed at it.

2. Discussions of both *noh* and *kabuki* are in: Bowers (1952), Ernst (1975), Brandon and Shively (1978), Hoff (1983), Gunji (1985).

3. The floating world is the term by which the popular entertainment district of Japanese cities is referred. In pre-Meiji Japan it included *kabuki* theaters and tea houses at which *geisha* performed.

4. Each school of *kabuki* choreography has a performance exam that when passed by a member of the school has allowed the dancer to perform under a name which incorporated the school's name into their own.

5. Kanriye Fujima taught in Spokane until 1991. She quit teaching in this community because she decided she would like to reduce her overall teaching responsibilities.

6. This pattern has changed during the years 1988, 1989, and 1990 as she has returned to Japan during the summer and fall to perform with the Hiroshima school.

CHAPTER III

THE MOVEMENT AND ITS AESTHETIC BASE

The direct antecedent of the movement vocabulary associated with *nihon buyo* is *kabuki*. However, *kabuki* during its evolution has assimilated into its performance vocabulary and associated aesthetic the performance forms that preceded it. Twentieth century *nihon buyo* incorporates elements of the entire history of Japanese dance theatre including *noh* and *bunraku*. Within its specific history it also involves the movement styles that are the result of stylistic innovations of its modern proponents. An understanding of the movement identified with *nihon buyo*, as Kanriye Fujima teaches it, includes an understanding of the general physicality of Japanese dance theatre, the movement style of classical *kabuki*, the movement qualities derived from *noh* and *bunraku*, the development of the movement vocabulary in the twentieth century, and its aesthetic association with zen philosophy and practice.

Basic Body Stance

The physical use of the body in *nihon buyo* varies greatly from the majority of western based forms. The fundamental difference is the dancer's relationship to gravity. The dancer in western theatrical and folk forms attempts to escape the force of gravity. Theatre forms of western dance (see Figure 3-A) consist of a series of movements that push into the earth in order to move away from it and its gravitational pull (ballet) or comment on the bodies relationship to the earth's gravity (modern dance).[1]

The purpose of dance in Japanese theatre is "to confirm the existence of the earth itself" (Gunji, 1970, p. 68). Comparing it to western dance Gunji states:

> Western dance is an attempt to express man's desire for freedom by striving to transcend the earth and escape into the universe. In Japanese dance, on the other hand, the dancer borrows the aspect of a god and hovers over the earth, blessing it and expressing love for it. (Gunji, 1970, p. 70)

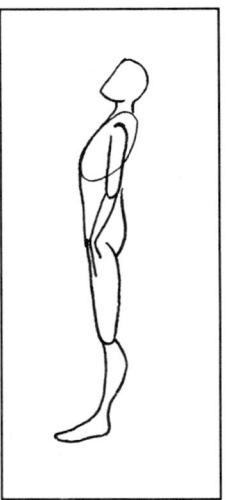

Figure 3-A

This close identification with the earth is an expression of the *kami* (gods) descent to earth to play in the form of dance. The Japanese theatre performer shares with other physical disciplines of Japan a body stance that keeps the energy focused on the center of balance in the lower torso (see Figure 3-B). In these disciplines the participant continually maintains a slight bent knee position while embracing the earth or in most cases the floor with the feet. The *buyo* interpretation of this basic stance includes the bent knee while maintaining a perpendicular line in the torso. Gestures of the arm and leg initiate the movement from one pose or posture to the next.

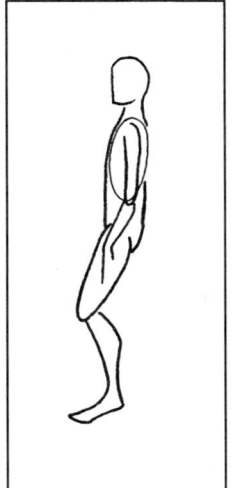

Figure 3-B

Despite the secularization of popular performance forms such as *kabuki*, Japanese theatre purports an emphasis on the spiritual dimension that is not necessarily found in western theatre.[2] This influences the movement style of the forms as they become symbolic representations of the continuity of tradition and by extension ancestors and age rather than of the future and youthful potential. Western dance forms seem to primarily concentrate on movements which require a strength and agility that can only be sustained until mid-life while Japanese forms focus on the development of spiritual beauty that comes through life experience, which young people do not possess. In comparison to western dance theatre, Japanese dance in general has a smaller more subtle movement vocabulary. Gunji attributes the spatial qualities of Japanese dance to a belief that the spiritual power of the dancer is intensified by generally being confined to a use of space that is limited by western standards. The western dancer uses the muscular energy in the torso and the appendages to extend the limbs into space and the Japanese dancer by comparison even in the most expansive gestures moves with limited spatial intent.

This general quality of *buyo* is characteristic of the three separate movement components associated with it; *mai*, *odori*, and *furi*. The term *mai* refers to the fluid arrhythmic abstract movements associated with classical forms of theatre such as *noh*. This theatre form evolved in the medieval period of Japanese history as the theatre of the samurai (warrior) class. Kan'ami (1333-1384) and Zeami (1363-1443), the father and son creators of the form, combined previous forms of theatre with aesthetics adapted from the court life and zen philosophy. The form, as they created it and as still presented today, has as its base song and dance. Many dance phrases are abstract depictions of the images created by the vocal accompaniment. The abstract gesture language associated with *noh* is often augmented by the use of the fan.

A good example of *noh's* movement style is *suriashi* or basic traveling movement. The dancer realizes this step with an erect torso, knees slightly bent and feet in parallel. With the help of the wooden floor and the sock like *tabi*, one foot slides forward with the majority of the foot pressing into the floor as the toes slightly release from the floor to aid in pulling the foot forward. With the body's weight centered in the pelvis, the forward step on one foot is repeated by a forward step on another. This basic step can be integrated with various gestures of the arm and head in locomotive sequences that move through the stage space in a variety of floor patterns.

Odori originated in rhythmic movement of festival dances. The original meaning for the *odori* was leaping as it referred to the quick change of feet in these communal festival entertainments. It has been refined by *kabuki* during its four hundred year history. As Gunji indicates:

> *Odori*, as we have noted, developed from the dances of the common people: the rustic festival dances called *bon odori*, the semi-religious *nembutsu odori*, and the townspeople's *furyu odori*--all group dances. The *odori* influence is most strongly apparent in the middle part (*nakaha*) of a dance number in which the characters perform a dance in unison, generally characterized by intricate hand movements. (Gunji, 1970, p. 76)

Gunji also refers to a custom originating in *odori* dances of individuals taking turns performing for each other at social occasions. The only phrasing similar to this in current *buyo* pieces, which may or may not be related to the initial custom, is the often repeated choreographic pattern of one dancer completing a phrase that is either echoed by or responded to by another dancer.

The third component is *furi*, or realistic pantomime. These movements are taken directly from the daily life of people and include the gestural style of different characters as well as the depiction of actions from daily life. Earl Ernst describes this highly abstract gesture language:

> Movement from real life is its point of departure, and *kabuki* dance reduces the multiple movements of human existence to their essential forms by narrowing, and thus intensifying, the visual impression of the movement, not by broadening it so that it no longer has precise meaning. (Ernst, 1974, p. 170-171)

The level of abstraction depends upon the character and the story depicted within the dance performance. According to Gunji there are many different kinds of *furi*. "There are many classifications of *furi*, from the extremely realistic *monomane-buri* to the abstract *fuzei-buri*. A particularly interesting type is the *ningyo-buri*, in which human dancers move in imitation of *bunraku* puppets" (Gunji, 1970, p. 76).

The enactment of the story associated with the movement of a particular character often requires that the performer manipulate one or more sets of properties (*kodogu*). These properties can vary from a long handled spear for a warrior to a silk scarf to enact a moment in a tea ceremony. However, the most common property is the fan (*ogi*). It can be used to illustrate a whole variety of actions from something as esoteric as viewing the moon, to more precise actions of playing the shamisen, drinking sake (Japanese wine), and cutting flowers. Many of the young *nihon buyo* students and all of the adult students own at least one fan with which they can practice. This fan resembles an actual fan used in performance in size and weight but it does not have the elaborate painted images of a fan designed specifically to be used with a particular dance piece.

Three Separate Movement Styles

The repertoire of dances which Kanriye Fujima teaches incorporates the components of *mai*, *odori*, and *furi* in three separate styles; classical, modern, and folk. The classical pieces are those most closely associated with *kabuki*. The three components of movement are interlaced in *kabuki* in a complex blend of movements that is almost always accompanied by a sung verse. The movement style is highly complex in its interrelationship between the movement which denotes a specific character type, the abstract gestures which convey the emotional state of the character, and the stylized gestures which illustrate specific tasks vital to telling the story of the song. In the development of the three in the enactment of a story the dancer moves from phrase to phrase in a series of gestures that incorporate primarily asymmetrical poses:

> *Kabuki* dance movement, though fluid and graceful, tends finally toward posture; its most significant moments are thus not realized in movement but in the achievement of a static attitude. The word used to describe the pieces which are primarily dance, shosagoto, literally means 'posture business'; and the dance resolves itself, in visual effect, into a succession of striking postures. (Ernst, 1974, p. 173)

Thus the dance is not always a moment by moment enactment of a specific set of sequential actions but often an attempt to recreate the feeling of a place or an event.

As mentioned previously the primary movement style of *nihon buyo* is based on that of *kabuki*. Kanriye Fujima refers to the dances and movement derived from *kabuki* as classical. This form of movement can be traced originally to the contributions to *kabuki* movement of the *onnagata* (men who play female roles) during the Genroku era (1688-1703). A. C. Scott (1955) explains the development of the dance pieces by *onnagata* as a method of increasing their roles in seventeenth century plays. The art of the *onnagata* is a portrayal by a male with a masculine physique of what, from a male point of view, is the ideal woman. Despite the fact that an actor of female roles will during the course of his career play women from a variety of backgrounds, he is still as Keene points out playing an abstraction of a type of woman. "The idea of the onnagata is an abstraction of womanhood rather than being a particular woman, and the superior *onnagata* imitates the *onnagata* of the past and their traditions rather than the behavior of real women" (Keene, 1973, p. 14). Nevertheless, the representation must also be recognizable as female to the audience. The *onnagata* is aided by stylized costume and make-up, but in order to be successful, he must also possess beyond experience and skill, a certain degree of charm and sensual appeal.

Famous *onnagata* of the Genroku period (1688-1704) included Segawa Kikunojo I (1693-1749) and Yoshizawa Ayame (1673-1729). As *onnagata* of the Genroku era, they were assisted in their portrayals of women by a change in traditional Japanese costume. Women's *kimono* sleeves became almost a yard long, while the *obi* got longer and wider. The *onnagata* used this exaggerated nature of the costume to help hide their obviously male physique and to emphasize the beauty of the character portrayed by a male body dressed as a female.

Since the Genroku period the *onnagata* have developed dances called *michi-yuki-mono* (travel pieces) telling the story of a journey. The *onnagata* also adopted plays from *noh* in creating such pieces as *Shakkyo* (Lion Dance) and *Kyoganoko musume dojo-ji* (Woman at the Dojo-ji Temple). These pieces were always accompanied by a *joruri* (ballad singer) who sang the story accompanied by a *shamisen*.

Beyond the innovations of the *onnagata*, the movement style of the *kabuki* was influenced by its competitor at the box office, the *bunraku* (a twentieth century term coined for the puppet theatre). The *kabuki* theatre began borrowing stories from *ko-joruri* or puppet theatre starting with the demise of the boys' *kabuki* in 1652. Beginning with the Genroku Era, there was a constant battle for audience between *ko-joruri* and *kabuki*. The *ko-joruri* began to replace *kabuki* as the most popular theatre in Japan. This was particularly the case after playwright Chikamatsu Monzaemon moved from writing plays for *kabuki* to writing plays for *ko-joruri*. (Gunji, 1985)

In order to remain competitive the *kabuki* companies adopted popular elements of the puppet theatre. This inevitably created drastic changes in *kabuki* that affected all levels of production. A primary influence on the movement style was the adoption by *kabuki* of a style of music called *gidayu bushi*. The music, originally intended for the short quick movements of the puppets, defined the movements of the actors. The *kabuki* movement vocabulary assimilated the puppet movement style in pieces originally derived from the puppet theatre. One of the famous *ko-joruri*-derived pieces has been *Yagura oshichi* (Oshichi at the Fire Tower).

Regardless of whether or not they include movement based on puppet characters, the movement of the *onnagata* or female character is spatially focused inward. (see Figures 3-C and 3-D) This inward pose is accomplished by a combination of a stable torso and a highly exaggerated inward turn of the leg which begins at the hip and ends with the feet in a pigeon toed position. To develop the capacity to maintain this essentially awkward hip-knee-foot position, some teachers require that their students keep the inner thigh and knee in constant contact. This focus is reinforced by a limited spatial use of the arms and an indirect focus of the head. The elbows are always kept close to the body as the dancer moves in a series of postures and gestures that move in and out of an asymmetrical line of the body. Except when manipulating a prop of some sort, the hands are often kept hidden within the sleeves of the kimono or placed in very specific poses. As mentioned previously, this convention was created by the early *onnagata* performers to hide their overlarge hands.

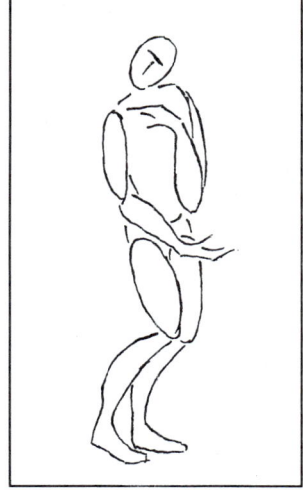

Figure 3-C

These generally light and indirect movements can be observed in the entire movement vocabulary of female characters. The characters walk by gently holding the weight over the back foot while the toe of the moving foot is brought forward still preserving the inward position of the foot and then lightly placed on the floor. Meanwhile, the same shoulder as foot releases slightly downward and the head moves in the opposite direction. To kneel, which in Japanese theatre is the basic sitting position, the dancer slowly lowers herself to the floor while still keeping her knees together and placing her hands with fingers held together in their lap.[3] This basic movement vocabulary associated with women characters can vary depending upon the character's age and position in society.

Beyond those pieces that focused on the lives of women, created for the *onnagata* actors, there also evolved *aragoto* and *wagoto* styles which focused on the physical representation of male characters. *Aragoto* style was the creation of Ichikawa Danjuro or Danjuro I (1660-1704). This physical style was expanded and extended over the years, primarily by his direct descendants. In plays which incorporate the *aragoto* style, the lead male actor is the center of attention. As Kominz points out:

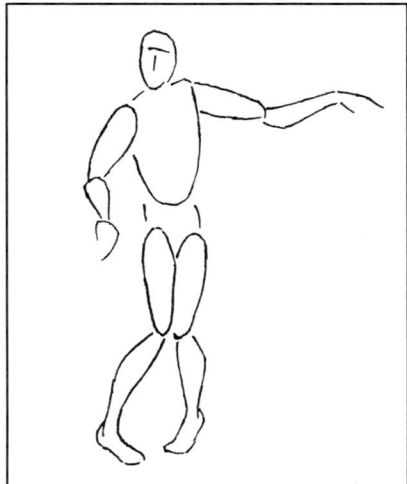

Figure 3-D

> The other actors, the words and music of the play, and even the gorgeous sets fade into insignificance; their role is to reinforce the image of strength and valor presented by the *aragoto* character and to bring the virtuosity of the main actor into clear focus. (Kominz, 1983, p. 347)

The movement associated with the *aragoto* roles is a complex interrelationship between a series of gestures and poses that illustrate the dialogue of the play. This set of character gestures often culminates in a final pose called a *mie* which incorporates both body and face. This facial grimace is to indicate heightened emotion. The entire movement vocabulary of the *aragoto* character is physically opposite of the *onnagata*. The movements are expansive with an external spatial orientation. The basic stance is an erect torso with knees bent and feet turned outward from the hip. Prior to actual movement the postural stance of the *aragoto* character resembles a dancer in the demi-plie position of ballet. With a series of strong direct foot and arm gestures the character strides through

THE MOVEMENT AND ITS AESTHETIC BASE 43

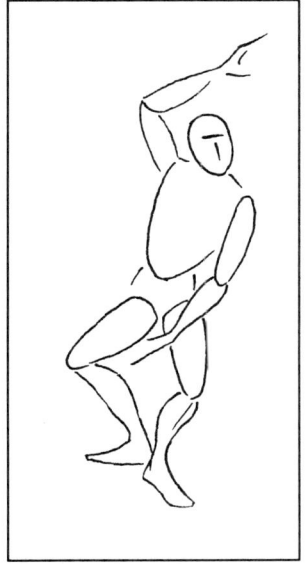

Figure 3-E

space while consistently maintaining a lowered torso by keeping the supporting leg bent. The associated gestures move away from the body in an exaggerated series of poses that illustrate the story and emphasize the effect of the costume. (see Figure 3-E and 3-F) When kneeling/sitting the *aragoto* character sits with knees apart and hands on his upper thighs. This position, as in the walk of the *aragoto* character, is the opposite in spacial quality of the characteristic inward knee position of the *onnagata* character.

The *aragoto* character has as its supplementary male character the *wagoto* (man of gentle business). Kominz suggests that the roots of this style are to be found in the *keisei kai* scenes of *women's kabuki*:

> *Wagoto* scenes included brothel scenes, lovers' trysts, and scenes of heightened emotion between family members or lovers. Various terms were used to describe kabuki's emotional scenes: *nuregoto* ("damp business", referring to weeping), *kagegoto* ("shadow business," referring to love in the shadows), and *keiseigoto* ("courtesan business," love scenes with courtesans). The term *wagoto* refers to these scenes as well as the subdued somewhat effeminate acting style employed by actors who played the roles of young lovers. (Kominz, 1985, p. 168)

The most famous *wagoto* actor was Sakata Tojuro (1647-1709), who played such famous roles as Izaemon, the sensitive amorous young lover of the courtesan Yugiri, in *Yugiri's Farewell New Year*. He was an advocate of an intuitive acting technique in which gestures were not formalistic but came from the inner feeling of the character. His approach to acting may have been the result of his lack of skill as a dancer. (Kominz, 1985) The physical style he originated is a middle ground between the physical style of *onnagata* and *aragoto* characters. The basic stance incorporates the turned out position of the feet with a gestural style that is more rounded and less direct than the *aragoto* character. This is partly accomplished by

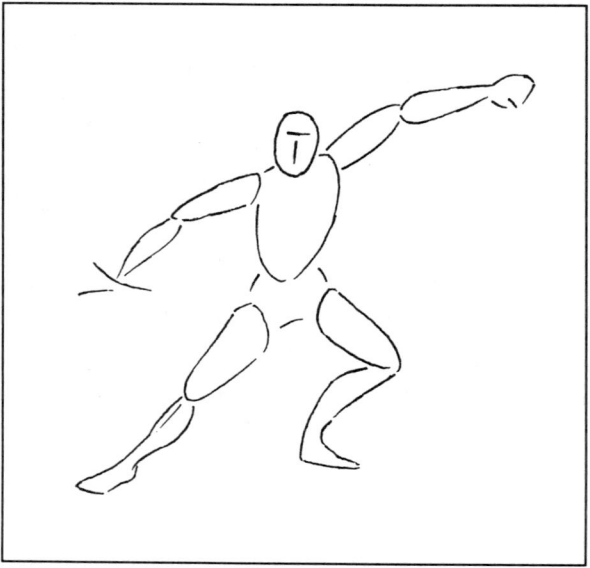

Figure 3-F

bringing the torso forward as you move carefully placing the weight on the ball of the foot first as opposed to the full foot of the *aragoto* walk.

In the realm of the classical style there are also characters that represent the townspeople of the *Tokugawa* period. These characters follow the general movement outlines established for male and female characters with appropriate adaptations depending upon their occupation. The movement for the individual character is reinforced by the props associated with the character.

The dance plays or *shosagoto* of *kabuki* can be divided into *henge mono* (general transformation pieces that require numerous costume changes), *soga mono* (dances revolving around the Soga brothers legend), *michiyuki mono* (travel pieces), *dojoji mono* (pieces revolving around the Dojoji priestess legend), *ishi-bashi mono* (lion pieces), *matsubame-mono* (pine tree or *noh* and *kyogen* pieces), and *sanbaso mono* (congratulatory pieces). Although the performance of *Kabuki buyo* is a highly refined technical skill, the goal of the performer is not to celebrate the physical body but to enact a story:

> It is important to remember that *shosagoto* is not just a display of technical virtuosity. The dances are not expressing abstract themes therefore, the dancers are characters in a story, there is dramatization, and all of the movements, however stylized, are rooted in reality. The creation of the fiction of the story and the technical skill of the dancer are admired equally by the audience. (Johnson, 1974, p. 50)

A second group of dances is referred to as modern to indicate their development in the twentieth century. These pieces, even modern adaptations of classical pieces, are more accessible to Kanriye Fujima's average student than those derived from *kabuki*. The modern pieces incorporate music by popular singers combined with classical instrumentation from *noh* and *kabuki*. One good example is *Hanafubuki dojoji*, a variation of the *kabuki shosagoto* piece *Musume dojoji*. The dance begins with music and movement style derived from *noh*. After the first few measures, the music changes to a modern orchestration which combines violin, *shamisen*, and a female vocalist. The movements are a combination of movements from classical pieces and those created in the modern *nihon buyo* style. The change in the musical accompaniment creates a slightly different use of the body line. The knees are not as bent as in other styles. Body postures and associated gestures are lengthened, thus creating a longer body line than found in the classical pieces. Gestures of the arms have a tendency to reach further into space. The dancer is less likely in these pieces to incorporate the intricate use of the kimono sleeve in ways that hide the hands. The timing of the dance also changes, as the modern music often has a consistent underlying rhythm for the dancer to follow, unlike the classical pieces which rely on the free-flowing voice of the singer.

The third group of related dances are the folk pieces which are refined versions of *minyo odori* (folk dances) of festivals from various regions of Japan. The movement style is similar to that of *obon* dances presented each summer in many Japanese American communities in the United States. The movement phrases often mimic the work life of farmers, loggers, and other laborers. The least choreographically complex of the three styles, these pieces usually (unlike either modern or classical pieces) begin with a movement phrase which is repeated symmetrically and returned to again and again. As is true of folk dances in any country there are folk pieces which have been specifically choreographed for the stage and feature difficult physical feats. *Tsugaru jongara bushi* (A

Rhythmic Tune from Tsugaru) performed at the 1990 recital was such a piece. It combined a lively folk song from Tsugaru in northern Japan with each of the six dancers controlling five separate fans. The dancers moved in unison to the music as they maneuvered the fans in and out of a series of tableaux.

Any dance regardless of type is made up of a series of movement phrases or *kata*. There are some *kata* that refer to fan positions such as *nigiri* (moving the fan in front of the body); *kaname* (holding the fan at the center); and *hiraki* (opening the fan). Other *kata* refer to specific ways of walking including *osuberi* (a sliding motion of one foot away from the other which may be accompanied by a variety of arm gestures); *mawari kaeshi* (a lift of the leg and a half turn followed by two steps, another lift of the leg, and a second half turn); *keri dashi* (a foot manipulation of the long kimono used for specific roles). Still others refer to gestures of the upper torso as does *sasu* (to point with one arm while bringing in the other arm). The combination of *kata* changes with each dance. People who have been students for many years learn new *nihon buyo* pieces relatively quickly as they are familiar with the standard *kata* for different movement styles.

The Dance's Aesthetic Goals

The student of *nihon buyo* is not only learning a set of movements. She is also participating through movement in a set of aesthetic ideals that reflect the centuries of evolution of Japanese culture. The primary influences have been shintoism, zen philosophy as it has developed since its introduction to Japan, (Suzuki, 1959) and the theatrical theory of medieval *noh* playwright, Zeami. Although many scholars trace various attributes of current theatre to their roots in any one of these elements, my focus is on the experience of the performer and the interrelationship of these as a part of the student's participation in the form. Therefore, this discussion will try to consider the aesthetic concepts as they are learned as part of the somatic training of the student.

As previously discussed, *nihon buyo* is taught not as in most western disciplines as a series of disparate parts that are delineated verbally and then regrouped to form a whole. Dances are taught as total entities.[4] The student imitates the teacher's movement until with repetition, the movement becomes ingrained in the student's body. Throughout the entire learning process, there is an emphasis on nonverbal, intuitive learning. The teacher will rarely explain a movement to the student. Instead, students are encouraged to develop increased levels of somatic awareness and to literally 'think with their body.' In this *nihon buyo* shares a similarity with Japanese physical disciplines in general. In these systems the student is expected to invest their total "physical and mental powers to unceasingly struggle for the solution to a problem" (Schmidt, 1986, p. 72). Kyoto based teacher Kansome Fujima, of the Kanjuro branch of the Fujima school, has referred to the learning process as deriving information by diligent application of the mind and body as a unit to the problem.[5]

This approach to teaching, which has many variations in different Asian physical disciplines, is used in Japanese society to encourage students to increase their level of mind/body introspection. With its roots in zen practice this level of introspection and mental exorcism through physical means pushes the student into greater levels of self awareness. The students are expected to constantly examine the reason for the organization of their learning process by the teacher. As Schmidt elaborates:

> Introspection allows critical examination of one's innermost self, one's emotions and beliefs, one's center of *kokoro* (heart) as it is known in Japanese, for the purpose of bringing about a harmonious ordering of one's actions with one's beliefs as well as those of his or her social nexus. Mental exorcism is another facet of self-cultivation that is concerned with inner purity and is not considered complete unless it eliminates all inner anxieties and frustrations which prevent the mind-body complex from functioning in a natural way. (Schmidt, 1986, p. 70)

The belief is that self-actualization is a result of understanding the body's existential existence in the world. A student who pursues one of the arts, including *buyo*, enters a path of study (or in Zen terminology a way) with a teacher who serves both as interpreter and transmitter of the techniques and philosophy of the tradition. The teacher then becomes the guide in the student's process of self-actualization and the study of the art becomes the means by which the self-actualization is achieved. "The underlying belief is that through concentration one can achieve anything one undertakes" (Lebra, 1976, p. 163). Despite the variety of different reasons the student has for the initial involvement in lessons, once involved in the teacher-student relationship, the student engages in an interaction with a teacher who will encourage her to discover unconscious fundamentals of self. The student who studies many different artistic paths finds that while there may be overlapping aesthetic goals each has its individual manifestation.

One of the primary architects of Japanese theatrical theory and its associated aesthetics was Zeami (1364-1444). In his writing, Zeami described both the creation of a method for training performers in a physical theatre and the primary aesthetic expression identified with it. (Rimer and Masakazu, 1984) The training of the *noh* performer was in nine stages of increasing development referred to as the nine stages of *hana* (flower). The ultimate goal of the performer was to be the stage embodiment of the aesthetic construct *yugen*.

Yugen has a long and complex history. It appeared first in Buddhist literary work of the eighth and ninth centuries (Tsubaki, 1971). By the twelfth and thirteenth centuries it had become established as an aesthetic value connected with court poetry (Izutsu, 1981). Zeami adopted *yugen* from the court society as an ideal that would help him to unify the dramatic form he was in the process of creating. The term has two components:

> *Yu*, the first component of the word *yugen*, usually connotes faintness or shadowy-ness, in the sense that it rather negates the self-subsistent solidity of existence, or that it suggests insubstantiality, or more accurately the rarefied quality of physical concreteness in the dimension of empirical reality. *Gen*, the second component of the word, means dimness, darkness or blackness. It is the darkness caused by profundity; so deep that our physical eyesight cannot possibly reach its depth, that is to say, the darkness in the region of unknowable profundity. (Izutsu, 1981, p. 27)

Zeami's early approach to *yugen* centered on unifying it with other ideals of the *noh* theatre such as *monomane* (imitation of things) and *hana* (flower) into a concept of "the beauty of gentle gracefulness" (Tsubaki, 1971, p. 55). His original approach, adapted from the life style of the court, was modified over time and the concept enlarged. The version of his old age incorporated the idea of *sabi*, "The concept at this ultimate stage was identified by Zeami with various terms, including *sabi* (the serene simplicity of the aged or the feeling of tranquil loneliness). The creation of this new idea resulted in the expansion of the 'realm' to the 'world' of *yugen*, as it were" (Tsubaki, 1971, p. 55). Zeami stressed that the training of the student to perform as an expression of either *yugen* or *sabi* should be through physical rather than conceptual learning. As Yuasa points out:

In order to grasp the mind's authentic mode of being, we must first reverse the ordinary view that puts the mind before the body, and place priority on the form of the body. Only then can one seek the authentic or essential mode of the body. Only then can one seek the authentic or essential mode of which we call 'mind.' For the true mind, that is the mind of the flower, is attained anew only via the comprehension of technique (*waza*), the body's correct form (*katachi*), through its training (*keiko*). (Yuasa, 1987, p.107)

Toshihiko and Toyo Izutsu applying a phenomenologist perspective to the work of Zeami include a similar perspective in their discussion of the aesthetic theory of *yugen*, "We may safely assert that *yugen* is not only an aesthetic idea or ideal but also an indication of a reality actually experienced by poets and artists as they focus their consciousness on that particular aspect of the phenomenal world" (Izutsu, 1981, p.27). Accordingly, the artist through the contemplation of the practice of the art expands her ability to experience the sensory world. The result is the development of internal psychic of the student:

Yugen, then, is the beauty not merely of appearance but of the spirit; it is inner beauty manifesting itself outward. The emphasis on inner beauty, as against the beauty of the outward appearance, is inevitable so long as the imitation in the *Noh* is of the inward spirit, of the true intent. It is the beauty of the inner most nature of things, the beauty of hidden truth. (Ueda, 1967, p. 60)

This inner beauty is developed through somatic experience. "It is a beauty of spiritual aspiration and yearning motivated by the desire to have sensuous images of the non-articulated, non-sensuous reality of eternal silence and enigma in the midst of the phenomenal world" (Izutsu, 1981, p. 28). *Yugen* in its contemplation of *mu* or nothingness is the foundation for all other Japanese aesthetic concepts that are part of the "Japanese art-theory, called *gei-doh*, namely, the aesthetic Way" (Izutsu, 1981, p.28).

In the study of an aesthetic way, such as *nihon buyo*, students learn to actualize *yugen* through the physical manifestation of the form. This is accomplished through the student's development of self-actualization through contemplation of the form that comes through participation in the study of it. A principal aesthetic concept associated with *yugen* is *ma*. This is the integration of time and space into the harmonious flow of the universe. *Ma* is silence within a flow of sounds and emptiness within a flow of visual stimuli. It is both a means of sensing the moment of movement and a pause in the movement. *Ma* is the expectant stillness of the moment preceding a change. The student is guided by the teacher to a somatic understanding of *ma* or the time/space continuum through an intuitive process which requires that the student focus her entire somatic awareness during the learning process. This is the opposite of most western style training programs which concentrate only on the use of the visual and auditory senses.

Other aesthetic concepts associated with *ma* are taught in the same manner. The most important to dance theatre is *utsuri*, or the moment nature is transformed, a transition from one state to another. (Gunji, 1970) In movement terms, *utsuri* can be either a transition from one body part to another, such as a foot movement to a hand movement, or it can refer to a change of mood and character within the dance. It reflects the Japanese belief derived from Buddhist philosophy in the constantly changing nature of existence. A momentary pose, such as a *mie* or facial pose from the *aragoto* acting style, is followed by a transition into the next movement. Zeami reminds *noh* performers of the importance of keeping the intensity of the mind in these moments:

> At the moment when the dance has stopped, or the chant has ceased, or indeed at any of those intervals that can occur during the performance of a role, or, indeed, during any pause or interval, the actor must never abandon his concentration but must keep his consciousness of that inner tension. It is his sense of inner concentration that manifests itself to the audience and makes the moment enjoyment. (Rimer and Masakazu, trans. 1984, p. 97)

Other aesthetic ideals associated with *nihon buyo* that are referred to by Masakatsu Gunji (1970) in his discussion of *buyo* include *kakucho* or rank and style. This refers to the level of spiritual development of the dancer or the ability to transcend her humanness that is displayed in her performance. This term is related to *okisa*, or "breadth of expression and depth of content," (Gunji, 1970, p. 71) which connotes not larger movements on stage, but the appearance from the audience's perspective of spatial depth brought about by a preparatory movement of the dancer. Each movement of the body is preceded by a movement in the opposite direction. The movements of preparation cause the performer to pause for a moment as they prepare in one direction to move in another direction. This preparation and pause causes the audience to concentrate on the movement and to see it as larger than it actually is.

Finally, Gunji indicates that unification of technique and spiritual development is referred to as *iki* (spirit). This artistic expression is associated with a way of life in general, that is, the ability to combine one's artistic life with one's personal, private life:

> No matter how much mechanical technique is added or how cleverly the dance piece is put together, technique alone will never produce true dramatic power. It is only when the various techniques are brought together in organic, artistic time-space, through an all-embracing, raw, spiritual strength, that living, full-rounded dance is born. (Gunji, 1970, p.71-72)

In the ultimate performance the self actualized dancer moves to illustrate the story in a set of movements which have become so ingrained in the musculature that they are accomplished with ease and without thought.

From the perspective of phenomenology, Izutsu elaborates upon the three levels with nine developmental stages of training identified by Zeami to accomplish a state of 'no mind.' While Zeami describes these stages in metaphoric terms and Izutsu in phenomenological, I would argue based on my observations from training both dancers and actors that the state of 'no mind' is a result of the somatic training of the musculature. Concentrating on the three larger categories or levels, one can consider the student's attainment of 'no mind' via muscle acceptance of the movement style or form. Within the first level, the performer moves first from cognitive existence to synchronic awareness of the dynamic tension of existence. The dynamic tension of the first level is the result of the muscular tension and often unnecessary muscle contraction associated with the uncertainty of newly acquired movement. In the second level the performer moves from contemplative awareness to focus the harmonious state of nothingness. This takes place as the student solves the tensions in the musculature associated with the vocabulary of the movement, uses less muscle contraction to achieve the required movement, and as a consequence feels more comfortable.

The experience for the performer is as if the movement is arising from the muscle without mental contemplation of the physical act as if from nothingness. This allows the performer to concentrate on the performance as a state of its own which leads to a synthesis of experience by the performer of the performance itself. This level is followed by a third level in which the performance acts as an entity of its own without conscious contemplation by the performer. There is a unity of somatic experience for the performer as the performer and performance become one. The performer portrays the physical representation of the character and the ideals of the art form she has internalized.

Students who learn a physical form through a method of training which causes them to incorporate all their sensory apparatus in learning the form participate mentally, according to Japanese philosopher Yasuo Yuasa, on both the bright and dark plains of consciousness. The bright level is the conscious level of experience. The dark level is the level of experience that is similar to the functions of the autonomic nervous system. It can also be considered to approximate the views of the lived experience of the body of Merleau-Ponty, Bergson, and the no-mind of Buddhism. Psychologists might refer to it as an aspect of the unconscious.

It is this dark level of consciousness that Yuasa believes the method of teaching proposed by Zeami is training:

> Initially, the body's movements do not follow the dictates of the mind. The body is heavy, resistant to the mind's movement; in this sense, the body is an object opposing the living subject (*shutai*) mode of being. That is, the mind (or consciousness) and the body exhibit an ambiguous subjective-objective dichotomy within the self's mode of being. To harmonize the mind and body through training is to eliminate this ambiguity in practice; it amounts to sujectivizing the body, making it the lived subject. This is a practical, not a conceptual, understanding. Although we tend to forget that which is cerebrally understood, we do not forget what we learned through our body. What we acquire through our body can be unconsciously, naturally expressed in body movements fitting 'form.' The 'mind' here is not the surface consciousness, but is the 'mind' that penetrates into the body and deeply subjectivizes it. (Yuasa, 1987, p.105)

The student of a Japanese theatre form is learning on two levels, conscious (bright) realization and unconscious (dark) knowledge. There are physical aspects to both levels. The student is physically conscious of the specific movement phrases as they are learned. As the movements become more ingrained they become part of the dark level of knowledge. As Mark Johnson illustrates *In the Body in the Mind* referred to in Chapter one, the student is learning on both levels through the congruence of the interaction of the body in mind a set of metaphoric understandings referred to often as culture. On an unconscious level these understandings influence her psychophysical approach to life. An example of this phenomenon is the experience of the student of zen meditation. The student of zen is consciously aware that she is sitting for a period of time in a physical posture allowing the mental images to flow through her mind without attachment or judgement. She is also, however, on an unconscious level through the daily practice of the sitting posture teaching herself to take a non-dualistic psychological perspective in relationship to life experience.[6]

When Kanriye Fujima arrived in the United States she brought with her not only her experience as a student in the *iemoto* within both the Yamamura and Fujima schools but the movement vocabulary and aesthetics that were part of the extensive history of Japanese theatre. Kanriye does not herself delineate as separate elements the system of learning, the movement components, and the various aesthetic principles. She teaches them to American students, as she states, by using the same methods her teachers used to impart to her both the dances and the personality influencing cultural values affiliated with them.

Notes

1. I have not included western folk dance forms in this discussion as this text focuses primarily on theatre forms.

2. Most histories of Japanese theatre trace its origins to the dance to entertain the sun goddess Amaterasu.

3. Despite the fact that the movement style was originated by male performers in Japan, the students in the United States are primarily female. For this reason I am using the feminine pronoun.

4. In order to continue the form, this style of teaching has been replaced in some places by a more western organized teaching style. A good description of a traditional method of teaching in *noh* theatre is Monica Bethe and Karen Brazell's article, "The practice of noh theatre," from *By Means of Performance*, New York: Cambridge Press, 1990: 167-193.

5. Personal communication July 1985.

6. A source that discusses the psychophysical influences of zen meditation is Suzuki (1959).

CHAPTER IV

THE STUDENTS

Although the majority of Kanriye Fujima's current students are Americans, they represent a diversity of distinctive life experiences. When Kanriye Fujima arrived in the United States in 1956, her first students included a small older group of *Issei* that was a combination of the early immigrant group and post-World War II immigrants, women who were known as *shin* or new *Issei*. There were also *Nisei* (second generation) and some *Sansei* (third generation) Japanese American students who ranged in age from grade school through junior high. Although her first students were a mix of all three generational groups, the majority of the students of the *nihon buyo* schools were female Japanese Americans. Recently, the interest in Japan reflected in the increase of Japanese language courses has also spread to the study of Japanese cultural forms. Over the last ten years, the student population has started to include students who are either members of interethnic families in which one parent is not of Japanese American descent or whose origins are in a completely separate ethnic group. The non-Japanese American students are generally students who are themselves or whose parents are interested in Japanese culture. The general population is however still primarily made up of female students. In the last four years there have been only three young men enrolled in the Portland and Spokane schools and none at the Ontario school. The students range in age from four to sixty, but most of them are currently in the four to eighteen-year-old age bracket.

In the last two years Kanriye Fujima's Portland area students have included college age students who are from Japan but in the United States to study English. While they are in this country, they are taking the opportunity to study *nihon buyo*. Their main reason for beginning study in this country is the financial accessibility of the form in comparison to Japan. As Atsuko Iwasawa explained, "I would have liked to study dance in Japan, but it is too expensive to study dance there. Here I can study and it is affordable. Also, I can perform the dances in this country without having to pay the large fees for performance they charge in Japan." These students add another interactional element to the school as they are not Japanese Americans but Japanese citizens studying *buyo* in America.

Besides generational, ethnic, gender, and age differences the students can be divided into those who have and those who have not become *natori*. The women designated *natori* are part of the complex *iemoto* system that is basic to Japanese culture and analogous to the traditional family unit as discussed in chapter 2. Because of Kanriye Fujima's certification and reputation within the larger Fujima School of Japan, the members of the Pacific Northwest schools have the opportunity to visit Japan to complete the performance examinations that will give them the rank of *natori*. This rank allows them to teach and perform under the school's name. Since Kanriye Fujima began teaching in the United States, five of her students, three from Portland and two from Spokane, have received this designation.

The process of becoming a *natori* represents a commitment by the women not only to study diligently with Kanriye Fujima in the United States, but also to travel to Japan for two months of the year in which they take the performance examination to study with Kansho Fujima, her teacher in Hiroshima. After this two-month period, they perform their two dances, a *matsu* (male) and a *fuji* (female) piece, just as Kanriye Fujima did for her examination, and receive their certification from the head of the school in Tokyo. The cost for each performer's certification is $10,000.

The students designated *natori* receive two symbolic indications of their affiliation with the school. One is the group portrait of themselves sitting with their teacher, their teacher's teacher, and the *iemoto* of the school. A second is the new name received by each student. This new name is a combination of the school's family name and the initial *kanji* of the *iemoto's* blended with a *kanji* chosen to represent them. For example, Kanriye Fujima is a blend of Kan form Kan'emon the name of the *iemoto* and riye. The last name is Fujima for the school. The students of Fujima Kanriye (written Japanese style with the family name first) or Kanriye Fujima (written American style with the family name last) generally list their names in programs in the American as opposed to the Japanese style.

Regardless of their personal background, female or male, Japanese American or Caucasian, each student refers to Kanriye Fujima in conversation neither as Kanriye Fujima nor as Madame Fujima, as she is sometimes known in the press. Instead, they call her 'Sensei.' And, each has a separate relationship with her 'Sensei' built upon the interchange that takes place in the individualized lessons. However all students have a personal history, a reason for the initial involvement in the study of *nihon buyo*, what they feel they gain from it, and how they believe it influences their lives. The individual nature of this experience is represented in the stories of the following five students.

Barbara Uyesugi (Kanhanae Fujima)

Nihon buyo is for Barbara Uyesugi a way of retaining a cultural tie with her birthplace, Japan. While she was growing up in Japan, she did not want to study *buyo* but instead concentrated on the piano. After she arrived in this country in 1948, she began to appreciate the beauty of the traditional Japanese art forms and began studying with Sensei shortly after her arrival in 1956. She is one of the few women who have attained the *natori* rank of the Fujima school in Japan, but she is also proficient in the art of *ikebana* (flower arranging) and is currently studying the *koto* (stringed instrument similar to a zither).

Barbara is the driving spirit behind the Portland based group Fujinami-kai. It is in her basement studio that Kanriye Fujima teaches each month when she comes to Portland. Barbara is also the primary organizer of the Fujinami-kai's many performances in the Portland area. As a result of her work, the Portland based school, Fujinami-kai, performs in Portland's Young Audiences in the Schools Program and recently won a performance grant from the National Endowment for the Arts.

With both a degree from Portland State University and strong ties to Japan through her family, she serves as a bridge both for non-Japanese trying to understand Japanese traditions and Japanese trying to understand the non-Japanese world. She maintains contact with the Tokyo dance world through her sister who is also a *natori*. Her house is often a temporary home for Japanese students who want to study English. She shares her knowledge of Japanese language and culture by teaching them in the Portland public schools. Recently with Kanriye Fujima's encouragement, she has started teaching *buyo*. Currently, she has six students who also take lessons from Kanriye Fujima when she is in Portland.

Barbara's approach to *buyo* is to acknowledge and embrace the depth of the tradition within which the form has developed. This includes the mutual obligation and respect between teacher and student that lasts a lifetime. She acknowledges that Martha Graham may think it takes ten years to make a dancer, but this is not true of Japanese theatrical forms. Instead, the student continues to add depth and skill with each passing year well beyond the first decade of study, or as Barbara quotes an old Japanese proverb, "You do not get old for nothing." Thus, her life and the dance are intimately connected, as she studies with Sensei both in Portland and in periodic trips to Ontario, arranges for performances, and serves as spokesperson for *nihon buyo* in the greater Portland area.

Nihon buyo and the tradition out of which it grew is, for Barbara, a great teacher in itself. Beyond the obvious skills associated with the dance, such as grace and physical control, Barbara believes *buyo* teaches other life skills. By being taught in a cultural system where many things are not explained orally, the students are forced to use their visual and kinesthetic awareness to learn. The result for the students is often an increased ability to focus their concentration on any subject they approach. Through the emphasis on the welfare or harmony of the group rather than the individual, the students develop sensitivity to the people around them. They learn to change their behavior in response to a personal need of someone else instead of being entirely concerned with their own desires and problems. The students also learn an appreciation for the past and the people associated with it in attempting to portray a variety of characters from different segments of Japanese history and society.

Barbara's personal life has not been without difficult adjustments. She lived through the war years in Japan, adapted to a new country and the related marriage as well as the death of her first husband and subsequent remarriage. Yet, these problems have never defeated her; instead, she has accepted them as part of a life fully lived and, as time allows her, has continued to explore and learn as much about both her adopted country and the traditional Japanese arts.

Miyoko Stroup (Kanhidemi Fujima)

Miyoko was born in Eharaki near Osaka, Japan. She and her family managed to survive the devastation of the war and the difficult times that followed by living with relatives on their farm outside of Osaka. It was then that she feels she learned the skills of survival and adaptability that have helped her adapt to life in the United States. It was also during this time she learned how to garden and how to teach herself to do things from the materials at hand.

For a short time following World War II, she worked for the city government in Osaka. However, her parents arranged for her to marry a Japanese American, and she came to live with him in Portland. She has lived in Portland since then, raising two daughters and investigating different aspects of her Japanese past from her home in the United States.

She describes herself as someone who sees something and then wants to learn it. With the aid of the local library she has taught herself how to make wine, to grow fruit trees, and to sew a *kimono*. These are useful skills for her life on her three acre farm in Oregon City, a community southwest of Portland. Her small farm has a variety of fruit trees and a large vegetable garden. Much of her time in the spring and summer of each year is spent growing and harvesting the many varieties of fruits and vegetables which she then preserves. When necessary she applies her ability for self-teaching to creating the necessary props for *nihon buyo* pieces in which she is performing. In 1990, she designed and made the masks for her character in *Oharame*.

Miyoko began taking lessons from Sensei in 1957 as soon as she discovered that Sensei was teaching. Miyoko would spend the day working in a garment factory and go from there at five to the studio where Sensei was teaching. The consistent lessons represented the fulfillment of a lifelong dream which started when she was in elementary school but had to be postponed during the war. The lessons helped to ease the loneliness she felt in a strange country where she did not speak the language. It brought Japan "close to her." When the only cheap transportation was steamship, the lessons made the physical distance that separated her and her natal family seem shorter.

Four years after she came to the United States, she gave birth to her first daughter and two years later to her second daughter. During this time, she continued to study, and each daughter, as she turned four, began taking lessons. Miyoko would take her lesson after her two daughters. This pattern continued for eight years but was stopped by a family crisis which forced Miyoko and the girls to give up their lessons. For the two daughters, this was the end of their study, but for Miyoko, the study of *buyo* was merely placed on hold. Several years ago, after her daughters had finished high school, she returned to study with Sensei and traveled to Japan in 1983 to pass the examination to become a *natori*. She has also started to study *shamisen* with Sensei so that she can better understand the music associated with the classical pieces of *nihon buyo*.

The earliest dances she remembers learning were female pieces such as *Harusame* (Spring Rain). She is still attracted to the classical, more formal, female pieces, but also enjoys the comic and male dances. Although she likes learning the male pieces, she does not feel that she performs them as well as female pieces because she is of short stature and it takes a larger physical presence to perform the male pieces. She plans to continue studying *nihon buyo* as long as Sensei is teaching.

The importance of *buyo* in her life has not diminished over the years. A portion of each day is spent practicing old and new *buyo* pieces. Another part is used in practicing the *shamisen*. Time is set aside each winter for a period of concentrated study with Sensei in Ontario. Each recital by the school incorporates her talents as a performer, costumer, and mask maker.

The function of *nihon buyo* in her life has not changed a great deal over the years. It still allows her to experience the depth of her Japanese heritage. Her recent visits to Japan, however, have convinced her that it is not a place she would like to live, as she feels it is too crowded and too noisy. She is content with a life that allows her to pursue her interests in traditional Japanese arts in an environment that includes clean air, quiet, and lots of trees.

Patsy Abe

Patsy spent the first eight years of her life on a truck farm outside of Gresham, Oregon, and her parents, as first generation Japanese Americans, did not have the money to spend on luxuries such as dance lessons. Patsy first studied *nihon buyo* when she was eight years old and living in an internment camp at Minidoka, Idaho. The lessons given in the camp were an opportunity she would not have had under normal circumstances. Time has erased the name of the teacher and the other eight-year-old friend with whom Patsy studied, but not the excitement of the lessons or of the performance given at the camp. Describing it as a pivotal event in her life, Patsy remembers "the beautiful costumes with wigs and pretty fan. I fell in love with the form as it made me feel connected to something good at a time when life was very difficult."

Despite the enjoyment Patsy derived from studying *odori*, she, like all the rest of the Japanese Americans, were anxious to be released from the camps. Following World War II, she and her family returned to the Portland area to rearrange the pieces of their lives. *Nihon buyo* was completely forgotten until 1965, when she attended a performance given by Sensei at a Portland high school. The performance reminded her of her experience as a child. Fortunately she was able to approach a friend who knew Kanriye Fujima and could ask permission for her to take lessons. She has been studying regularly since then.

From the very beginning, the pieces Sensei taught her have been a challenge that require her to concentrate simultaneously on a variety of information from how to use the fan to where her feet should be placed. Over the years she has evolved an approach to understanding Sensei's teaching that focuses first on the body and later on trying to blend the movements to the exact phrasing of the music. More recently she has begun to videotape her lessons (as have other students) so that she can use the tape to practice at home. This method has helped her to learn a variety of both male and female roles. However, she admits to finding the male roles more difficult than the female, as the stance and attitude of the characters seems awkward in comparison to the female.

The study of *buyo* is for Patsy another extension of her understanding of herself as Japanese, or as she puts it: "I love anything to do with Japan." Her home and life are a testament to this statement. Her ranch-style home is filled with Japanese art, from pottery to wall hangings. She is one of the few members of Fujinami-kai who owns several of the expensive silk performance *kimono*. She has studied the tea ceremony. She and her husband are active members of the local Buddhist church and the Japanese American Citizens League. Her son, while he was growing up, studied judo, while her daughter studied *buyo* prior to going to college. As an elementary school teacher Patsy shares her knowledge of *nihon buyo* and the tea ceremony with her students as part of their classroom work. She finds they are fascinated by the *kimono* and *obi* and enjoy the children's dances she teaches them.

Nihon buyo is such an integral part of her life that Patsy cannot imagine not studying it. She feels that Sensei has taught her through the form that it is possible to move effortlessly and that when one seeks to learn something one should do it with humility. "You can never do the dance perfectly. There is always something more to learn about the movement, the music, the character. There will always be something there to learn and Sensei will find it."

Diane Hinatsu

Diane Hinatsu is a third generation Japanese American whose family migrated to the United States from Fukishima, Japan, prior to World War II. Diane started taking lessons with her sister Michele when she was seven years old. She took lessons every day for one week a month while Sensei was in Portland. Her mother watched the lessons and took notes. During the three weeks between lessons she and her sister were expected under their mother's guidance to practice each day in the living room. She enjoyed the lessons until she was in junior high and then she became embarrassed by them. She was trying to understand herself and her place in the world and the dance classes didn't seem to fit the world she was in. It was confusing partly "because I felt as white as all my friends, but sometimes they would expect me to be different because I was physically different." The dance lessons just seemed to increase this confusion.

This was a confusion that resolved itself when she left the Portland area to go to college. She did not take lessons while in college but pursued her interest in dance through courses in ballet, modern dance, jazz, and other mediums. It was the interest in dance in general that helped her resolve her Japanese American identity. She began to appreciate that she lived in two worlds, each of which had a unique viewpoint. Now she lives in Portland and studies with Sensei but also pursues an interest in dance in general by performing with a local modern dance company.

As an adult studying *nihon buyo*, she feels particularly lucky to be studying with Sensei, who epitomizes for her the ideal of teacher and performer. As a teacher, she appreciates the patience with which Sensei has taught her over the years. "She is always so encouraging and integrates the movement of the lesson with the story it is based on. The classical pieces that are really difficult, and require a lot of subtle movement of the head and hands, are developed in a consistent process that allows me to learn them." When taking a lesson Diane tries not only to do the movements exactly as Sensei is, but to imitate the expression and feeling as well. Her experience has taught her that only in modeling Sensei completely so that her gestures perfectly match her will she learn the piece correctly.

Although Diane has studied many different styles from pieces based on folk forms to *onnagata* roles from *kabuki*, the most challenging are the female roles, whether they be traditional *kabuki* pieces or modern abstract performances. "The male roles are more like western dance in that they use more space and allow you to express yourself in big ways. The female pieces require that you express the same intensity of emotion, but you have to do so with much smaller and more subtle movements."

Diane believes it is Sensei's personal love of what she does that has encouraged Diane to continue studying. Associated as she has been with other dance teachers, Diane is sometimes amazed at Sensei's dedication, as well as her humility. "The performance is always created for the students for their personal growth. If it is necessary for her to take someone's place in a group piece due to illness, she does so even if it is a children's dance. She also makes sure that all of us have our costumes on and are ready to perform. She even stands outside the curtain and gives us our cues."

Diane is considered by Kanriye Fujima and other members of the school to be accomplished enough to become a *natori*, but for her, it is not a decision to be made lightly. Her hesitancy is a result of several factors, one of which is the tremendous cost. A second consideration is the increased responsibility attached to the position. She realizes from observing the other *natori* in the school the level of commitment expected. Until recently she has been uncertain as to whether or not she is ready to fulfill the obligations associated with the position. Encouraged by Sensei and the other *natori*, Diane has decided to prepare for the *natori* exam to be given in Portland the summer of 1993 during a visit of Sensei's teacher Kansho Fujima. Although not made easily, the decision is part of a redefinition of her life which includes marriage and the further embracing of her Japanese heritage. The only reason for not taking the exam at this time would be an inability to raise the $10,000 school fee.

Diana Snell

In the last ten years, there is a whole new generation of young Japanese Americans, *Yonsei* and others, who are being raised during a time of increased ties between the United States and Japan. They can take courses in Japanese language and culture at their local high school, community college, or university. News programs from Japan are beamed via satellite. Japanese films are featured at American art cinema. In the 1980s *sushi* became during a period of time the 'in food' of the upwardly mobile in many American communities.

Diana Snell was a sophomore in high school when I first met her. She and I became working partners in a classical piece, *Genroku hanami odori* (Cherry Blossom Dance) for Kanriye Fujima's thirtieth anniversary recital. Diana was born in Portland, Oregon. Her mother was born and raised in Japan, but her Scotch-Irish father was raised in California. Her family has maintained close ties with her maternal grandparents in Nara, Japan, a historic community located near Kyoto. When she was thirteen she attended the funeral of her maternal grandfather, who came from a line of Shinto priests that stretched back seventeen generations. Deeply impressed with the ritual, she decided she wanted to know more about her Japanese heritage.

When she went to high school, she enrolled in Japanese language and culture courses and has followed that course of study while enrolled as a student at a local university. Unlike many young women who stop taking *buyo* lessons once they graduate from high school, Diana has chosen to continue to take lessons and to perform regularly with other members of the school. As she has matured as a dancer, she has increasingly been given more difficult classical pieces to perform. She intends to study indefinitely with the goal of someday becoming a *natori*.

The most difficult part of studying *nihon buyo* for Diana is trying to bend her knees enough so that her slender five foot nine inch frame does not tower over the other young women with whom she is on stage. She will never forget how generous and supportive Sensei was when she grew six inches in one summer and was feeling tremendously awkward at her new height. Sensei made her forget her size by having her concentrate on the movement. "She constantly encouraged me in order to keep me from feeling discouraged. But she does that with everyone. She takes whatever skill you have and helps you make it better."

Diana, now a senior in college, still continues to study Japanese language, literature, history and *buyo*. She spent the summer after high school in Japan visiting relatives, improving her language skills and becoming acquainted with the country. The increased interchange between Japan and the Pacific Northwest provides her with many opportunities to continue to improve her language skills. She is uncertain where her emphasis on the study of Japanese culture will take her. But upon graduation she plans to work in the travel industry and to return to Japan to explore the history of the maternal side of her family and its connection with shintoism.

Larry Kominz

Larry Kominz, a Professor of Japanese Language and Theatre at Portland State University, was first exposed to Japan as a high school student living in Tokyo with his parents where he attended the local American School. Although his foreign language study at the time was in French, he did take a course in India and the Far East as part of his curriculum. The result was a fascination with the potential intermix of cultures that is so much a part of Asia. He continued this interest at Colby College specializing in East Asian Studies with an emphasis on Japanese language and culture. In 1972, he returned to Japan and gained his first exposure to traditional Japanese theater watching performances of *kabuki*, *kyogen*, and *noh*.

Larry began his first study of Japanese theatre techniques in 1973 with the study of mask making with Udaka Michishige of the Kongo School of *noh*. He followed this with three years of intensive study of *noh utai* (chant and song) and *shimai* (dance to vocal accompaniment), and *maibayashi* (dance to orchestral accompaniment). Having explored *noh* he decided to add *kyogen* to his repertoire of forms studied. He studied *kyogen* with the 'living national treasure' Sengoro Shigeyama, the *iemoto* of the Shigeyama branch of the Okura School of *kyogen*. Larry made his *kyogen* debut at the Kanze theatre in Kyoto in 1978 in the popular play *Kaki yamabushi*. In *kyogen* he felt he had discovered a form in which his facility with the Japanese language served him well in presenting the required comic vocal inflections of the *kyogen* actor. He felt lucky to be included in the circle of reliable amateur disciples of Sengoro and the opportunities this gave him to perform at the numerous shrine festivals in and around Kyoto with many noted members of the Shigeyama family including Sengoro's father Sangoro. Besides Sengoro was a wonderful teacher who made the learning process easy by his jovial manner which made you feel secure but still carried an underlying expectation that you would absorb the fine points by careful imitation of his voice and movement.

In 1986 and 1987 while acting as the resident director of the Tokyo exchange programs for the Oregon State System of Higher Education, he studied *kabuki* with Matazo Nakamura of the National Theatre Kabuki School. The lessons with Matazo Nakamura were brief as Matazo's schedule kept him moving from one city in Japan to another. When Larry returned to Portland in 1988 he made contact with Barbara Uyesugi and made arrangements to start taking lessons both with her and with Sensei. His first goal as a student was to learn a male and a female piece that he could teach the following summer at a workshop on traditional Japanese theatre forms directed by noted Japanese translator Thomas Rimer at the University of Maryland. Having succeeded in learning both *Oyagi* and *Kuroda bushi*, he concentrated on learning several classical pieces including *Goro*. In 1990, he appeared with the other members of Fujinami-kai in their spring recital performing *Goro* and *Byakkotai*.

Larry extends his interest and study of Japanese traditional theatre to modern fusionist productions which blend a combination of western and eastern performing techniques. During several visits to Kyoto, Japan he has worked with the NoHo Theatre Company on applications of traditional Japanese theatre techniques to the twentieth century plays of Yeats and Beckett. In Portland, he has worked as a dramaturg for a local theatre's production of *Rashomon* and an original worked entitled *The Passion for Fresh Flowers*.

Of all the forms he has studied *nihon buyo* is for him the most challenging as it requires a level of motor control and physical subtlety for which his language based academic training did not prepare him. Despite the frustration that sometimes accompany lessons, he truly enjoys the opportunity to be living and working in the Pacific Northwest and still be able to be transported back to Japan every time he goes for a lesson with Sensei.

Larry considers Sensei to be a master teacher of her form who is able to provide an atmosphere of quiet encouragement while still expecting students to be committed to perfection of the form. He appreciates the fact that she devises the lesson to fit the student always starting within the framework of their experience and building upon it. He observes that his relationship with Sensei is different from some of the students due to his fluency in Japanese and also his constant trips to Japan. This allows him to converse with her about areas of common interest not necessarily shared by the other students.

The satisfaction which Larry takes in his involvement in *buyo* and in other Japanese theatre forms is the potential acting range that accompanies the dedication of the individual to the form. "By eliminating myself and taking on the form, I can participate in the life of characters which are completely outside of the sphere of my normal life. I can be a *samurai* or a *geisha*. When people ask me how I as a man can create a believable female character on stage, I say that wasn't me that was *buyo*." It is this fascination with the form and the potential for continually expanding his understanding of Japanese culture through study of the form which will keep him studying traditional Japanese theatre indefinitely. He feels doubly lucky when, the demands of a family with young children do not allow constant trips to Japan, that he is able to take lessons with Kanriye Fujima as it continues what he experienced in Japan.

Other Students

Kanriye Fujima feels that the study of *nihon buyo* by students in the United States is a continuation of a trend started in Japan prior to World War II. According to her, girls from upper class families were encouraged to study *buyo* as part of their self development. As she puts it, "A girl was given dance lessons to teach her to be womanly, graceful, and poised." Susie Nishihara, Ontario resident and the mother of two daughters who studied with Sensei until they went to college agrees with her. But she also believes the dance lessons helped her daughters who were born in the United States to learn Japanese culture and manners. Other mothers of students give the same reasons as Susie Nishihara for having their children take lessons and stress the connection it provides with their Japanese heritage. One Portland resident who grew up on a farm thirty miles outside of Ontario observed, 'I never had the opportunity to study dance when I was growing up because we lived so far from town and therefore I felt cut off from some of my heritage, so I wanted to be sure that my daughter had the opportunity to experience Japanese culture."

This desire to understand their Japanese roots has been a reason cited by many women who study the form. Chisao Hata, an active member of the Portland arts community, informed a newspaper interviewer that when she was growing up she learned little about her Japanese heritage. "It was a personal interest of mine to get back to my roots. It was a part of myself I wanted to know more about. This type of dancing is helping me to do that. It makes me slow down. It's teaching me about another whole world that's a part of me." The desire to maintain ties with their Japanese heritage is also one of the reasons that both Barbara Uyesugi and Miyoko Stroup decided to become *natori*. Barbara puts it this way: "Growing up in Japan you take for granted art forms like *nihon buyo* and want to learn all about western things, but when you get to the United States and look at Japanese arts from the perspective of living here you begin to see how beautiful they really are and what important values they can teach you."

In conversations on what they learn studying *nihon buyo*, students regardless of background have stressed the importance of learning to better understand yourself and your position in the world by portraying different characters that are related to a specific cultural past. Their descriptions of *nihon buyo* also include the importance of being involved in a system of learning, the working with other people, and learning to be aware of other people's needs as well as your own. Kanriye Fujima herself does not discuss any of this as concepts; instead she relies on the faithful rendition of her own training to speak for her.

Despite the differences in background the majority of the students are Americans. As such, they bring to their lessons their particular personal cultural background that is a combination of social, family, and personal history. The students' statements seem to reflect the impact of their study of *nihon buyo* in three areas of their lives. First, the importance their study has had in their lives of giving them the opportunity to be exposed to some part of their past or to an intriguing culture from the other side of the Pacific. Next, the value discovered in engaging in the consistent discipline that is a part of a continuing study of the a Japanese artistic form. Lastly, the influence 'Sensei' has had as a teacher on their lives. Of the three, the last seems to possess the greatest meaning for the students. Her definition of teacher, evolved from a Japanese model of personal relationship between student and teacher, has generated a feeling of reverence for her.

CHAPTER V

THE STUDIO: THE PROCESS OF TEACHING

The process of teaching is a multi-level experience for the students that includes their interaction as part of the organizational hierarchy of the school, their individual exchange with Kanriye Fujima during lessons and rehearsals, and the performance of those pieces she has selected for them on stage. This discussion of the process will focus on the organization of the studio and Kanriye Fujima's approach to all students with examples of individual students.

The Organization of the School

Typically, students begin lessons at approximately age four (or five) and continue until they are eighteen or graduate from high school. Some of these students return to study *nihon buyo* once they finish college, but most do not. However, there are women, such as Susie Nishihara, who return to study *buyo* once their children leave home and their child-rearing responsibilities have diminished. The students Kanriye Fujima teaches fall into two categories: young people under the age of eighteen and women who are or could be grandmothers. The one group for which there are almost no students are women between twenty-five to forty.

Anyone interested in studying *nihon buyo* with Kanriye Fujima does not make arrangements with her to take lessons, but instead with the school or the group she has established in the community. Fujinami-kai in Portland and Fujihana-kai in Spokane operate as separate units, but each is associated through Kanriye Fujima with the Fujima School of Japan. Kanriye's teaching in Ontario is supported by Toei-kai, a group of forty families. According to George Iseri, spokesperson for the group, the Ontario club has been organized specifically to support *nihon buyo* and provide learning and performing opportunities for those who enjoy the art form.

Students who join a school are not subject to an audition. They are screened informally in the lesson itself for their interest and dedication. Students who do not practice are tolerated, but not necessarily encouraged. Each student who becomes a member of the *kai* (school), agrees to pay a $45 per month charge for lessons ($55 per month for *natori*) and a $25 annual fee each spring.[1] The annual fee covers the cost of the basic maintenance of the group plus the annual New Year's present to Kanriye Fujima.

The members of Fujinami-kai in Portland who are *natori,* and therefore the highest ranking members of the school after Kanriye Fujima (Barbara Uyesugi and Miyoko Stroup), have increased responsibilities for the continuity of the school and Kanriye Fujima's teaching. Examples of their responsibilities are varied. Kanriye, when she is in Portland, has for the past thirty years stayed at either Barbara's or Miyoko's home. When in Portland, she teaches in Barbara's basement studio. At any performance, whether it be a small one as part of a Portland international celebration or a major recital, they help Kanriye arrange the dress, make-up, and hair of the performers. They are also present in the studio during a major portion of the day when she is teaching in Portland. They help the young children into and out of their practice *yukata*, serve as additional members of a group piece if other performers are absent, act as models for the student's approach to studying the dance, help mend and repair costumes, bring cold or hot tea (depending upon the time of year) to Sensei and others in the studio, and fix meals for her.

The students are expected to follow the example set by the *natori* and commit themselves to a process of learning the dances in which all aspects of their education will be controlled by Kanriye Fujima. Barbara Uyesugi talks about the relationship between the student and the teacher that is part of the *iemoto* system as one of "a lifetime of mutual respect and obligation." She believes the selection of a teacher should not be a decision made in haste. As continued in the United States by Kanriye's relationship with her students, the teacher in the *iemoto* system is not someone that you take a few lessons from and never see again. Instead, there is a mutual responsibility between student and teacher. According to Barbara, this responsibility requires mutual sensitivity on the part of student and teacher. Or as she puts it, "There is a desire on both sides to communicate with each other." The teacher, in this case Kanriye Fujima, has responsibility to help the student to grow as a personality within the chosen form. The student's responsibility is to approach the teacher and the study of the form with humility and serious concentration.

The *natori* in this hierarchial system of responsibility are currently the organizers who insure the general administration and organization of the school. As they take on more of their own students, they continue to serve this function but also become the link between their students and Kanriye Fujima. A result of their teaching is the development of two categories of students: 1) those students who only take lessons from Kanriye Fujima; 2) those students who take lessons from one of the *natori* and also take lessons from Kanriye Fujima.

The Process of Teaching from Child to Adult

Kanriye Fujima has said both in personal conversations and in newspaper articles, "I have never given birth to children. But I have lots of children. All my students are my children." Notwithstanding the formality of *nihon buyo* tradition, there is a warmth and concern that exudes from Sensei towards each of her students. Her face breaks into a smile as each student comes into the door. She moves to help the student who may have momentarily misplaced the plastic sack of practice wear which is left at the studio between lessons. During the lesson, Sensei's tone and manner are soft and encouraging as young students try to remember the sequence of movements. At the end of each lesson, each young student is handed a lollipop as a mark of congratulations. When the teen-agers graduate from high school they each receive an appropriate gift, often jewelry, that signifies their new status as young adult women.

Sensei creates this environment of warmth and understanding even though she rarely speaks to the students in English. Although she can speak English quite well when necessary, all conversation within the studio before and during lessons between herself and the *natori*, or other students who can speak Japanese, is always in Japanese. During the actual lesson, there is only the occasional phrase or explanation in English. The *Sansei* mothers of students generally do not speak nor understand Japanese and are amazed at the ability of Sensei to communicate with their children. Each time Sensei is mentioned in a conversation, the mothers indicate their respect for her ability to teach the pieces without consistent communication in English. They often indicate their desire to be able to speak

Japanese. They seem to take pride in the fact that their children are learning from a woman who does. Kanriye's native fluency in the Japanese language validates her role as an exponent of Japanese culture in general.

Students encounter other barriers to learning beyond their inability to speak Japanese. The initial obstacle is the basic body stance which is the opposite of the movement style associated with their school physical education programs and other dance classes. A second obstacle is the music which accompanies the dances. Classical Japanese music does not follow conventional western time signatures, but rather the flow of the singer's voice. The student is faced with the two-fold dilemma of remembering movements that accompany lyrics she does not understand, and following unfamiliar rhythms.

The student is also trying to learn a dance about a subject which, for her, has no basis in past cultural experience. Regardless of their ethnic heritage the majority of the current students have never been to Japan. They have no knowledge of the Tokugawa period of Japanese history or of the associated *kabuki* theatre from which the movement style is derived. They may have seen a picture of a *samurai* or a *geisha* and have a vague idea of what the position of each held in historical Japan, but they have no idea of the attitudes and beliefs of either group or how they functioned in the society as a whole. As one student put it, "I am having a difficult time portraying a ferryboat man. I have never even seen one."

Sensei does not try to directly solve these problems. Instead, she relies on the method of teaching in which she herself was trained as the solution. Considering both their cultural and movement background, she constructs individual lessons which help the students to achieve specific personal goals that she has set for them. The private lesson between herself and the student varies not only according to age or experience but also with the personality of the individual student. While retaining an overall consistency, the lessons will vary from student to student both in the degree of complication of the movement phrases and the related cultural material.

By nine o'clock when the first student arrives, Sensei is waiting attired in traditional Japanese dress including *kimono* and *obi*. Each student comes a few minutes early to change from street clothes into a *yukata* and the special footwear, *tabi*, which help the dancer to create the smooth gliding walk associated with Japanese theatre movement. Once the student has finished dressing, she moves to the center of the studio space sitting on the floor in *seiza* waiting for Sensei to indicate she is ready to begin. Each student, regardless of age, then bows and says *onegai shimasu*. The lesson proceeds for the next half hour, Sensei tailoring the one on one lesson to fit the skills of the student. At the end of the lesson the student bows again and thanks the teacher. She takes off her practice attire. And as she was taught in one of the first lessons, she carefully folds her *yukata* before putting it away and leaving the studio.

The lessons are very different in teaching and movement style from western dance classes. The first major difference is the size of the studio space necessary for a class. Because dances do not rely on extended gestures of the legs or large combinations of the limbs and torso but on subtle gestures of the limbs including the head in relationship to the torso, the space required is much less than a western dance studio. The basement studios of Sensei in Ontario and Barbara Uyesugi in Portland are approximately 350 square feet. Of this space, there is only about 200 square feet available for actual lessons as the rest of it is taken up with storage areas filled with costumes and props. By comparison, the size of a modern or ballet studio would be closer to 1,000 square feet.

The lessons diverge from western classes not only in their individualization and size of studio, but also in their organization and length. In a western studio the group classes are generally an hour and a half in length. This time period is divided up between movement sequences to warm up the body at the beginning of the class that slowly evolve into longer movement phrases. The longer phrases require that the dancer move the length of the space available. The average lesson Sensei teaches is a half hour in length.[2] The entire time is spent learning the dances in their entirety, one phrase at a time.

If the student does not know the dance about to be taught, Sensei always begins by taking her through a small portion of the dance and repeating it several times, often singing the lyrics along with the recorded music. She sometimes gives brief instructions in Japanese to indicate a position of the foot or a movement of the hand and arms such as *hite* (back), *dashite* (front), *hidari* (left), *migi* (right) or *kurutto mawatte* (turn). She may indicate the timing of the dance with vocalizations such as "ching, ching, ching" which imitate the sound of the *shamisen* or "hup" to indicate the timing of a phrase. Other times, she will turn off the music and just sing the lyrics as she takes the student through the movements. She encourages the youngest children by telling them to turn their head toward mommy, or toward teacher, or to look at the doll or umbrella. If a child still has problems, she gently comes next to her and places the child's body in the proper three-dimensional pose that is so much a part of the *buyo* repertoire of movement. The dance is taught in this manner, portion by portion, until the entire dance has been learned.

A student of any age knows that she has passed to the next stage of learning when Sensei sits in front of her on a chair. At this point, she goes through the upper body movements as a reminder of the timing of the dance while the student performs the piece in front of her. If a student seems lost during any section, Sensei repeats it with the student again, but soon returns to her seat, only indicating changes in the timing. The final stage is reached when Sensei turns on the music and waits for the student to perform the piece by herself. During a lesson at this stage, the dancer performs the piece several times. At the end of the piece, Sensei makes any necessary corrections in terms of body position and timing or integration of the movement to the music. Because each dance piece tells a story, it is necessary for the dancer to move in relation to the *joruri* or singer. Therefore, the dancer, in order to perform the dance piece successfully, does not specifically memorize the music and lyrics, but must have enough physical awareness of them that her body responds appropriately.

The student, either young or old, is always first taught those pieces which Sensei believes will be closest to some familiar movement and frame of cultural reference. (For a list of most often taught dances see Appendix B.) New dances are added that progressively help the student to develop certain character traits. This is an intuitive process conducted by Sensei and sometimes seems to include an element of trial and error. Occasionally, she will begin to teach a dance, and, then move quickly on to another because she realizes that the dance is not appropriate at that time for that student.

The organization of the student's learning and performing is completely controlled by Sensei. It is she who chooses the dances and the order in which they will be taught. This is as true for the *natori* as it is for the beginning student. A student may desire to study a specific dance but understands that Sensei decides if it is appropriate for her. It is an aspect of her teaching that is never discussed among the students, nor in the case of the younger students, among their parents. It is an unstated rule that everyone accepts. The result is that students of all ages, with the exception of the *natori*, often do not know the name of the dance they are in the process of learning or why they are learning this particular piece. Unless they speak Japanese, they may not know the meaning of the words to the dance until the final stages of learning it. The student of Sensei must suspend all questions associated with the words "what" and "why" and accept her authority completely. During the many hours I watched her teach in Portland and Ontario, I never saw a single student or parent question her authority.

Regardless of her students' ages, Sensei seems to sense the long-term and short-term mental state of each of them. A student's lessons will never be mechanically repeated but varied in content depending upon the student's ability to concentrate in general and to concentrate on a specific dance piece. Concentration or focus is one of the personal abilities she values most in a student. One method of increasing the student's concentration is to expect them, even when they are just observing, to watch quietly another's lesson rather than visit with fellow students.

While participating in a lesson, the student is expected to follow the total movement and repeat each segment to the best of her ability. If she is having problems concentrating during that particular lesson, Sensei may suggest that she stop a few minutes between segments so that the student can "think it through in her head." Another tactic Sensei might employ is to repeat the movement phrase over and over again in rapid succession. A third teaching strategy is to add another section of the piece. This gives the student who may be having problems with the previous section something else to focus on. When all other methods have failed, Sensei will simply end the lesson early.

All children, no matter how young, begin learning dances that require them to use some form of prop, usually either a doll, parasol, or fan. These can be used in a representational manner, for example, a child using a *kasa* (umbrella) to protect herself from the rain, or in an abstract manner to depict a specific image. For example, a fan is often used to portray different elements of nature, including different phases of the moon, falling cherry blossoms, etc.

The dances for beginners have been short pieces in some way associated with the lives of children. For instance, in *Ningyo* (My Favorite Doll), the song told the story of a little girl playing with her favorite doll. This was one of the first pieces that I watched five year old Jodi learn. Using a cotton-stuffed doll for a prop, Sensei maneuvered Jodi through the song's refrains which describe the difficulty the girl has in deciding which *kimono* and which *geta* (wooden shoes) she should put on her doll. Even though she had learned the dance the previous month, Jodi kept forgetting the sequence of movements related to the section of the song in which the girl pretends the doll is crying and tries to put her to sleep. Sensei kept repeating the section over each time using a different strategy. She moved from sitting in front of Jodi to illustrating the movement with hand gestures, to getting up and doing the movement with her, to using simple verbal cues such as "look at Mommy" and "look at the doll," and finally, to adjusting parts of her body to correct a pose. As Jodi appeared to remember the movement, Sensei sat in front of her again and together they repeated the dance.

Another early dance for young children is *Hanakage*. A parasol is used as a prop and the story is of a small girl hiding beneath the flowers. The parasol represents the flowers. Two other examples of dances for children between the ages of four and six are *Kami ningyo* (A Paper Doll) and *Otsuki sama* (Mr. Moon). *Kami ningyo* does not use any props but does require that the young dancer learn to manipulate the sleeves of the kimono in a number of ways to tell the story of a paper doll who goes out in the rain and gets wet but hates to take her medicine. *Otsuki sama* is in honor of the moon, a common motif in many Japanese songs and dances. The dancer uses a fan to tell how youthful the moon looks year after year. It never grows old, although it does change. When it is crescent-shaped, it resembles the arched eyebrows of her beautiful sister, and when it is full, it resembles the lovely bouffant hair-do of a beautiful maiden.

With these dances, Sensei introduces the child to various facets of the *buyo* vocabulary in a manner she can incorporate and build upon. To accomplish this, Sensei frequently uses songs sung by children in simple two-four time. The movement phrasing for the majority of these beginning dances is less complex than later dances, and has numerous symmetrical repetitions. There is also a tendency to repeat a movement or a step four times rather than three times, as in the dances learned by teen-agers and adults.

In all the early dances the primary character is a young girl portrayed through stylized walks and poses. These walks and poses stress two primary characteristics of the female *buyo* character: the pigeon-toed walk and the S-shaped curve of the body. The female movement style is also found in the movements of the head--nods and shakes as well as the beginnings of the three-part head movement or *mitsu-buri*. In this intricate neck movement, the dancer turns her face to one side, tilts the chin to the same side and then following a curve of the chin tilts the head to the other side. During the movement the eyes are slightly anticipating the movement of the head. All head gestures are integrated with simple gestures of the arms and hands. These are sometimes combined with stamps and quick changes of weight.

The child is also introduced in these early dances to the basic floor patterns, the diagonal and circle. For example, a parasol is placed on the floor and the dancer makes a circle around it, or a fan is placed downstage and the dancer, balancing on one foot on every third step, makes a circle upstage, returning downstage to the fan. The child's tendency to move in parallel lines with the front of the stage is slowly shifted to a focus on the diagonal with Sensei's repeated gentle adjustments of the child's body. Sometimes as a child assumes an incorrect physical position, Sensei readjusts her head, turns her torso or changes the position of her arms and hands so that she is placed in the aesthetically correct pose. This gentle manipulation molds the child's body to the correct form so that she will be able to repeat the position naturally and without effort.

The constant adjustment of the body into what seemed to me to be artificial poses reminds one of the adjustments that are made in the development of a bonsai or the placement of flowers in an *ikebana* arrangement. Each section of the body is, as is a bonsai tree, reshaped with each new pose that is introduced. The movements between the poses are considered to be the path from one image to the next. The final product, either a bonsai tree or a dance, are according to one Japanese teacher of the form, Kansome Fujima, considered to be a natural imitation of nature.

As the dances become more difficult, there are larger movement combinations involving upper and lower parts of the body that the dancer must learn to integrate. In the children's dances, these phrases are indicated within the song either by vocal or rhythmic stress. In teaching *Kami ningyo*, a dance which has one difficult phrase that requires a quick change of the feet in a total count of five beats, Sensei first takes the child through the phrase as part of the entire dance with the music. She repeats the phrase several times without the music, counting it out in Japanese and English. The music is then put back on and the entire section repeated.

Each child is allowed to progress at her own speed, with new dances added according to individual learning ability. At any one time most children are learning two dances, each about five minutes in length. Each piece stresses different aspects of the form. At the early ages, this usually means either two different kinds of props or a dance with a prop and a dance which focuses on the use of the *kimono*. Beyond the specific movements, Sensei seems to focus in the lessons for the youngest children on increasing their ability to concentrate. The length of the phrases presented increases with the child's ability to remember larger amounts of somatic information.

About the age of six, most children have also started to learn dances which focus on various aspects of Japanese culture. *Kawaii sakanaya san* (A Little Fish Vender) is a piece about a fish vender walking around the town to sell fresh fish. The child, carrying a fish basket as a prop, illustrates with explicit movements the life of the fish vender as the singers sing:

How do you do?
Would you like some fish today?
No? Then I'm on my way to another house.

I have all kinds and I'll cut them to size.
Well, I've sold all my fish for today.
Thank you all and I'll see you tomorrow.

The children also start to learn various festival and folk dances from a variety of parts of Japan. These dances combine information about Japanese culture with stories that have universal appeal for children. One often-taught piece is a festival dance *Bura bura bushi* (Festive Dance of Nagasaki). It tells the story of a girl who is out for a stroll during festival time. She meets many people in a gay, holiday mood. One of them is a drunkard who goes staggering along the road. As the girl continues her walk, it begins to rain so she protects her head with her apron. The strap of her wooden clogs breaks and she limps hurriedly home. Each movement of the story is illustrated by using the *kimono* to represent articles of clothing and gestures of the hands and feet to indicate the problems of breaking a strap on a shoe while walking home.

The movement vocabulary continues to increase in complexity with each added dance. There is less and less repetition of basic movements and more development of phrases in which basic movements are linked together to form longer phrases. There is an increase in the integration between the *odori* or rhythmic sections of the dance and *furi* or mimetic sections. The student dancer begins to develop a kinesthetic awareness of the extension of the movement into and out of each pose and relies less on the pose itself. In recent years, some parents have started to bring video cameras with them to the studio so that they can film the dances their children are learning. The taped dance is used by the child as a reference point from which to practice during the three weeks a month Sensei is in another community, and the four winter months when Sensei is not teaching.

As the children move into the upper levels of grade school, the dances continue to incorporate ideas and symbols associated with historical Japan. *Kikuzukushi* (Chrysanthemum Dance) is one of the most popular of these pieces. It has been performed repeatedly at programs of the different schools since 1959. The young girls in the piece wear hats that resemble the national flower of Japan, the chrysanthemum. As a group they move from pose to pose in a variety of tableaux. Another dance that incorporates Japanese symbolism is *Harusame jishi* (A Lion Dancer in the Spring Rain). This is one of the numerous dances that feature the lion, as a symbol of endurance, strength, and good fortune. The story portrayed is of young professional entertainers who are performing the lion dance for crowds of people at a spring fair on a rainy day.

There are also several dance pieces which emphasize the different roles of women. Some pieces concentrate on the role of women as entertainers. In *Maisugata* (Portrait of a Dancing Maiden), a young girl is studying the art of dancing and gives up all other personal desires to do so. *Maiko* (Dancing Girl) is an often performed piece about an apprentice *geisha*. The dancer begins the piece standing facing upstage while twirling a translucent stage umbrella. She turns and moves the umbrella to illustrate her presence in the beautiful scenery of Kyoto. In one of the more complex sequences of *kata* taught to young dancers, she replaces the umbrella with a fan. This is used in conjunction with the umbrella in a series of poses that combine the two props with the dancer in a symmetrical tableaux. The piece ends with the dancer delicately holding the umbrella and using a series of tiny steps to run off stage. *Fuji no hana* (Wisteria Blossoms) is one of a series of pieces that uses the wisteria, the crest of the Fujima school, as a metaphor for a graceful woman. *Fuji no hana* which expresses the essence and beauty of this flower is usually the first of several pieces of this thematic material that a young dancer learns.

The students continue to learn a combination of classical and folk pieces as they progress from grade school into junior high. A common theme connecting the two age groups is baby sitting. *Komori* (The Baby Sitter) is an example. With a baby tucked into the back of her costume the dancer incorporates the use of a pinwheel in series of gestures and poses as "one of the many girls who came from the Niigata region, on the Japan Sea coast, to work in Edo (old Tokyo) as nurse maids. The nurse maid looks at a mountain off in the distance and it reminds her of home. She fantasizes about future love and marriage for herself and for the girl she is baby sitting.'[3] A variation of this theme is the group piece *Itsuko no komori ningyo* (The Baby Sitter Doll). A poor village girl is hired out to a wealthy family. She goes out to play with a baby strapped on her back and is teased and taunted by the other children. Her clothes are shabby, she is treated badly, and she is very homesick.

As the students become junior high age the dance pieces become increasingly complicated both in movement style and in the number of props. The phrases become longer and more intricate with fewer symmetrical repeats. Many dances incorporate the manipulation of more than one prop within a piece. The dance will open with a dancer using a fan and end with her using a branch of flowers, or it will begin with just a manipulation of the *kimono* and later incorporate the fan. The group pieces also continue to involve interrelationships between the dancers both in poses created by a group of dancers and in assorted character types within the same piece.

The lion is the focus in *Echigo jishi* (Lion Dancers of Edo) a duet for two dancers. This is an adaptation of Utaemon Nakamura III's 1811 adaptation of *kakubei jishi*, the traveling lion dancers of the Echigo Province. The original dancers "wore a colorful costume, with a bizarre lion mask over their head and brandished a peony branch, while beating a small drum attached to their chest" (Scott, 1955, p. 98). The face of the dancer was visible, as the mask was fastened to a silk crimson canopy worn over the head.

The dance created by Utaemon Nakamura III used the costume of the *kakubei jishi* in a three part portrayal:

> The first part portrays a dancer on his way to the big cities, wearing the mask, beating his drum and carrying a peony branch. The second part gives variations on the gay movements of the Echigo dancer who has by this time discarded mask and drum. The third part does not actually concern the lion dancer, but depicts a village maiden washing clothes in a stream, thus bringing into play a dance accessory known as a *sarashi*, a strip of white cloth more than three yards long and a foot wide, mounted on a grip which is held in the hand. It is manipulated to form figures while dancing and finds a parallel in the scarf dance of the Chinese theatre. (Scott, 1955, p. 98)

Scott's description of the *kabuki* version of *Echigo jishi* could be a description of the dance piece performed by teen-age students of Kanriye Fujima. It has been a part of performances since the first recital in 1958.[4]

As teen-agers, Kimi and Michele were taught this piece. By the end of the dance, the dancers were manipulating the long white ribbons in various related patterns. During a lesson prior to the 1987 recital, Michele and Kimi were rehearsing this piece in costume. This was a difficult piece to practice in the small space of Barbara Uyesugi's basement studio as the long ribbons kept getting caught in light fixtures, sections of the costume, and other people. Sensei kept repeating the dance adjusting problem segments. As they found becoming continually entangled in the ribbons enormously ridiculous, Michele and Kimi kept repeating the same movement errors over and over again. Eventually, Sensei stopped the practice laughing at herself and the students and suggested that everyone have some cold tea and then repeat the dance. This strategy was successful as Kimi and Michele were able after the short rest to actually find a way of using the ribbons in the space without incident.

Students of high school age are expected to be able to perform with ease the basic postures associated with female characters. They are also expected to be comfortable with a constant bent-leg stance and movements which require that one come from *seiza* to a standing position easily. This age group is often taught numerous classical dances on the theme of being a Japanese woman. Often these pieces incorporate all the movement phrases learned in past pieces and apply them in more complicated combinations. *Rokudan* (Dance in Six Parts), a dance in six separate sections, using a single fan, two fans together and a *fukusa* (silk cloth) used in a tea ceremony, is a good example. This piece combines the variety of ways of using both the fan and the *fukusa* to enact the extensive training a young woman of high social standing must undertake to learn all the arts associated with social graces: the tea ceremony, flower arrangement, and calligraphy. Beyond the varied *kata* this is one of the few dances that relies completely on non vocal musical accompaniment of the *koto*. A student who has come to rely on the voice for changes in the phrasing must now apply that kinesthetic knowledge to a single instrument. The student who has developed over the course of the lessons both a high degree of kinesthetic sensitivity to the music and muscle memory of the *kata* makes this transition with relative ease.

Other dances that focus on female characters are *Genroku hanami odori* (Cherry Blossom Dance), and *Hanami dojoji* (Flowers of Dojoji). These dances are set in the Genroku Period of Japanese history and describe young women dancing in the spring under the cherry blossom trees, viewing the flowers in the garden of the Dojoji temple, and as *geisha* dancing under the cherry blossoms. In portraying young women the students are required to practice the exaggerated slow, sustained, pigeon-toed walk of a woman. The entire gesture language is restrained with arms rarely reaching above the head or extended away from the body. The head is in constant motion moving in subtle gestures to illustrate the mood of the character.

As the students reach junior high and high school age, their mothers are less likely to be at the lessons than when they were younger. Also, girls this age are likely to come to the lesson with a greater number of mental distractions due to the escalated complexity of social and emotional relationships natural to this age group. Their ability to concentrate on the lesson is often diminished in comparison to younger students. But after years of lessons, their knowledge of the vocabulary of *kata* is greater. Sensei modifies her approach with these students, often teaching longer sections of the dance but repeating the dance with them more often. She also begins to increase the number of modern pieces that they learn.

The dances to modern Japanese music differ from the classical dance pieces in the general line and style of the movement. They do not require the knees to be nearly as bent nor the feet to be turned in to the same degree which creates a longer body line. The popular music, to which the dance is created, is similar in structure to popular ballad music in the United States. The singer repeats verse and refrain to music in a regular rhythm. The dance follows this pattern with movement phrases being repeated rather than constantly evolving into a new set of patterns. The underlying beat does not allow for the sustained pauses and associated poses as does the arrhythmical structure of classical music. Therefore, the modern dances have a sense of constant flow without the extended pauses that are an integral part of classical *buyo*.

The change in movement style is not necessarily accompanied by a thematic change. Women in modern ballads such as *Taki no shiraito* (A Taisho Ballad) are portrayed fulfilling their duty even at cost to themselves. In *Taki no shiraito*, a female musician falls in love with a poor student and provides the money for him to finish school by borrowing money from a loan shark. Later in life, the student becomes a judge, and the woman who helped him financially is brought before him for her dealings with the illicit money lender. Despite the fact that he convicts her, she is happy because of his success.

It is important to remember that, unless it is translated for her, the typical student does not understand the words sung by the singer. Her interpretation prior to performance of the song is based almost entirely on her interaction with the movement and the music. The first time she actually learns what the words to the music mean may be at the time of the performance either in the program or through a program announcer. The more complex the story the more difficult it is for the student to understand it due to her lack of cultural knowledge. Sensei approaches this lack of cultural knowledge by teaching the dances in a sequence that begins at the simplest level, easily accessible to the student, and adds complexity as the student matures as a performer. Additionally, Sensei tries to solve this problem by explaining the meaning of the dance or the story line to the advanced student. For instance, in teaching Diane Hinatsu the modern piece *Agari sai no hana*, she first teaches most of the movement of the piece to her and then explains the emotional tone. "It is a soft dance because of the sexy nature of the male singer's voice." Finally, she translates the basic meaning of the words telling Diane that the singer is comparing the person he loves with a flower.

Among the high school students, there is the occasional student such as Diana Snell. Diana pursues her interest in her Japanese heritage beyond lessons with Sensei to classes in Japanese language and history within the local public school system. (The classes would not have been available within the public school system to her parents.) The lessons become an opportunity for these students to practice their language skills. Barbara and the other *natori* encourage them by speaking to them primarily in Japanese and by correcting their errors in grammar and pronunciation.

It is only as the student is nearing the end of high school that Sensei begins to teach her the difficult classical pieces developed from the *kabuki shosagoto* pieces of the *nihon buyo* repertoire. These usually include a piece such as *Fuji musume* that incorporates the use of the long floor-length *kimono* which trails behind the dancer as she moves. At this stage, the dancer is believed "to be formed" so that her feet will stay naturally in a turned-in position. What she learns at this point is to manipulate, using the *keri dashi* technique, the long *kimono* in a manner that appears graceful.

The student, who studies beyond high school, begins to learn the congratulatory or ceremonial dances that are the standard pieces performed at the beginning of a *nihon buyo* program. There are a variety of these dances, many related to the *sanbaso* pieces that begin *kabuki* performances. The dance was originally borrowed by *kabuki* from *noh* drama. In *noh*, it goes under the title of *Okina* and is "a sacred dance always performed at the very beginning of the main performance; its purpose was to pray for the peace of the world and the safety of the realm, as well as good harvest" (Scott, 1955, p. 89). In *kabuki*, it is the opener of the November performing season. The purpose of the dance at the beginning of the program is to clear the air of evil so that good luck will prevail throughout the performance. There are several different *sanbaso* pieces performed, including *Ayatsuri sanbaso*, in which the performer emulates the movement of a marionette. Other pieces use other symbols, such as the imperial household and the chrysanthemum (*Kiku no sakae*), the pine tree (*Matsu no miodori*) or the ocean waves (*Shinyoku ura shima*) to create images of harmony, long life, and happiness. A complicated piece *Shochikubai* (Pine, Bamboo, and Plum) featuring three solos by separate dancers combines the pine, bamboo, and plum imagery with joyful scenes from Japan's holiday celebrations. The congratulatory dances are considered difficult for three reasons: first, they combine almost all sections of the *buyo* vocabulary; second, they often require the performer to play both male and female roles within the same piece; and third, they often require the dancer to execute a gliding *suriashi* step from *noh* that appears simple but is actually difficult to accomplish with the appropriate ease and smoothness.

Beyond the congratulatory dances, the persistent student begins to learn more and more pieces that require a more sophisticated level of characterization. These dances are often taken directly from kabuki as in *Musume dojoji* (The Lady of the Bell). This dance is considered one of the most difficult of the repertoire as it requires a series of props and costume changes. The main character is a beautiful girl who experiences the joy of falling in love and then the anguish of unrequited love. The dancer is expected to physically through the *kata* portray the emotional life of the character as she slowly transforms herself from a beautiful maiden to a demon. To be able to enact this complex role the student must have, beyond a well developed knowledge of the *kata* and sense of timing, an ability to portray through a series of subtle postures and gestures the nuances of the emotional life of the character. This requires the student be cognizant of the connection to the torso of gestures of the head and limbs. An ability referred to in western acting terminology as subtle energy transformations or transferences. This increased level of sensory capability is necessary as the student cannot depend upon facial gestures, as one does in most western based theatre, to convey the emotional transformation of the character. Although helped to some extent by costume and prop changes, the metamorphosis of the character is depicted entirely from the alterations of the physicality of the dancer.

Another set of dances prompts the student to develop male characters that repeatedly include the legendary *samurai* Goro who, with his brother Joro, seeks revenge on the men who killed their father. These dances focus on a body posture opposite that used in the female pieces. Instead of being turned in, the feet are turned out. Instead of focusing inward toward the torso the movement focuses outward away from the body. And instead of relying on small subtle movements of the arms and hands close to the body, abstract and mimed gestures are used which require especially bold movements. The student has been prepared for the potentially difficult transition from female to male posture by the combination of folk dance pieces using the male posture and female characters that the children have learned from the beginning. Two popular dances which focus on the Goro character are *Ame no goro* (Goro in the Rain) and *Goro tokimune* (Goro, the Samurai). Other male characters are part of stories of a husband and wife team of vendors as in *Yoshiwara suzume* (The Bird Vendors of Yoshiwara) and in *Tamaya* (The Bubble Vender).

The dancer at this stage also learns pieces that require the use of masks, as in *Mitsumen komori* (A Baby sitter of Three Masks). A baby sitter tries to make a baby stop crying by telling a story using three separate masks. The story is a familiar one of two men and one woman. The woman prefers one of the young men and the other becomes jealous. With the help of a stage assistant the dancer begins the story with one mask, and then changes from one mask to another as the story unfolds. In this and a similar piece *Kagura men* (A Comic Dance of Three Masks) there is an emphasis on the comic aspects of the characters. The choreography requires that the dancer highly exaggerate the accepted conventional movement style of both men and women by enlarging all the movements.

The dancer at this stage is familiar with the specific *kata* of *buyo* that are combined to form a dance piece. Sensei will often use the Japanese term for the *kata* as she teaches the dance. A student who has studied with Sensei for many years recognizes these *kata* as extensions of the movements she began learning when she was five.

The students of Sensei agree with Gunji and others (see Chapter 3) who have suggested that the movement of western theatre dance concentrates on presenting the possibilities inherent in a young body. The majority of western dancers quit performing when they arrive at middle age because they can no longer perform with the level of physical skill as when they were young. The opposite is true of Japanese theatre dance. The more experienced dancers frequently repeat with a sense of satisfaction an old Japanese saying: "Art has a beginning but no ending-- pursue it for a lifetime."

The Adult Dancer

Adult students fall into two categories: 1) continuing students who began when they were young, quit at some point and are now returning, and 2) those students who did not have lessons as children. In either case they are treated differently from children, being expected to put on their own *kimono* and *obi* without help and to remember more of a dance piece at any specific time than the children. This latter expectation varies with the experience level of the dancer. An experienced student is expected to learn the dances faster than others, as they already have a larger vocabulary of movement. A *natori* is expected to be able to recognize the dance vocabulary or *kata* in Japanese. Sensei will, when teaching one of them, say the name of the *kata* as she is teaching the dance. The *natori* are also the only students permitted to join another student during her lesson. They stand on either side of the student taking the lesson so that they can refresh their memory of dances they have already learned. At the end of each lesson, all students including the *natori* kneel in *seiza* and say thank you in Japanese.

The initial lessons of the new adult students proceed at the same pace as that of a young teen-ager. They do not begin with children's dances, but with pieces that reflect their past experience. For instance, training for those dancers who have some western dance training and are accustomed to turned out feet and large body movements often begins with a relatively simple male piece called *Kuroda bushi*. Using a spear and a fan, the dancer enacts the movements of a samurai warrior. Sensei's goal is to have the students begin with those dances which are easily physically accessible. As a male member of the Ontario Japanese American community described it, "Sensei teaches people to become the most they can, both as dancers and as individuals."

A woman who does not have a background in dance might begin with what is called a tea dance, a short five minute piece that incorporates imatative gestures taken from movement style associated with the lives of women, i.e. cutting and arranging flowers or serving tea. Later, she might learn *Harusame* (Spring Rain), a dance about a *geisha* who gazes upon the plum blossoms glistening with raindrops and the humming birds singing after a spring rain. Another possibility would be *Kurokami* (Raven Hair) which portrays the life of a professional entertainer.

Even for the students who begin dance training as adults, the process that Sensei uses to teach them does not vary from that she uses with children. She teaches them at the speed in which, in her judgement, they can absorb the information. (Some experienced students learn two five minute pieces in five days of half hour lessons.) The older student is usually taught more complicated pieces as their bodies begin to assume naturally the correct posture for the repertoire. The older students are also taught with a level of verbal communication that does not exist in the lessons for younger students. This communication takes the form of short sentences in Japanese referring either to the name of the individual *kata* or the direction and quality of a movement.

The atmosphere of the studio during lessons of the older students varies from strict attention to relaxed horseplay. One morning I was the first student to arrive. I was learning a difficult piece entitled *Matsu no midori*. I had learned the piece to the point that Sensei would sit out sections of it and watch me go through it, only making a move when I had forgotten what came next. Miyoko, as *natori* are allowed to do, had come down to the studio to join the lesson and was standing to my right, going through the piece as well. Periodically, I would get frustrated when I could not seem to coordinate a movement with the timing of the music.

My tendency was to use my peripheral vision to try and see if Miyoko knew the phrase. After several false starts, Sensei stopped me, saying, "Miyoko does not know this dance. You do. If you try to follow her, you will certainly be wrong. She is learning it from you." Chastised, I began the dance again but this time relying on myself and my knowledge of the dance. Later, Sensei and Miyoko told me not to become too frustrated because that was the dance used for the Fujima school examination and had all the basic *kata* in it. Miyoko encouraged me by saying, "Once you have learned this piece well, all the other pieces would be easy."

Once I had completed my lesson, Barbara and Micki began going through the piece that Barbara and Diane Hinatsu were going to perform for the American College Dance Festival. Sensei kept having them practice the entire dance because they were finding the intricate timing of some sections difficult to repeat correctly each time. Miyoko and I sat and watched quietly. As I sat there, I thought how often I had been at these lessons and how quietly focused Miyoko and the other *natori* were on the lessons of the other students.

Moments later, Sensei suggested we take a short break. We began talking about how the *Obon* dance *Nihon no obon* sounded like a popular rock and roll tune. Barbara said that it reminded her of the music the instructor had used for the social dance class she had taken once. She and Micki began comparing mambo and rhumba steps, laughing as they watched themselves in the mirror. Sensei watched us with a smile on her face and with a slight nod of her head indicated it was time to continue with the lessons.

Micki's lesson was next. She was learning *Ame no goro*, a *shosagoto* piece from *kabuki* about a warrior who takes revenge on his enemies. It is a difficult male role that demands the dancer be able to perform both male *aragoto* and *wagoto* styles. Sensei stood in front of Micki with Barbara standing slightly to the side and went straight through the entire fifteen minute piece twice. Micki then asked a couple of questions about foot placement and immediately started rewriting sections of her personal notation.

What is Learned

Sensei works intuitively to help the students learn personal qualities she believes will make their lives easier. This teaching is not restricted to the dances taught in the lessons of the student but through the totality of her teaching relationship with each of them. This includes the organization of relationships within the studio and inherent adherence to respect for hierarchy and tradition associated with the *iemoto* system in which she herself was trained and has utilized in her teaching in the United States. Students have an opportunity to observe communication styles among Sensei and the *natori* which rely more on subtext than verbal codes. Through the combination of observation and interaction they participate in the concept of *giri* or social obligation. They observe the *natori* accepting their position within the hierarchy of the school and completing the obligations to their teacher, school, and art form. They in turn are expected to fulfill their obligations associated with their position which include attendance at lessons, participation in performances, and continued support for the school as adult audience members.

Although Sensei will sometimes explain the story line of a piece to the student who does not understand Japanese, her primary method of teaching is to perform the dance while the student attempts to copy every detail of Sensei's movement with her own body. Sensei will adjust the body of the student to the correct posture only if the student can not seem to translate Kanriye Fujima's movement correctly on her own. She does not attempt to gain the correct placement of the student's bodies by talking about line, shape or extension. The emphasis is on the complete and total imitation of one person by another using primarily nonverbal methods of communication.

This approach is the antithesis of western based education as it relies on nonverbal means to teach basic concepts. Instead, she moves the student through a set of dances she believes will teach, within the movement structure of the dance, the appropriate concept. For example, students are not told that one of the goals is for them to learn inner strength which is manifested according to Sensei in an ability to completely concentrate on a task. I had a tendency to anticipate a movement and thus move too quickly from one *kata* to another. To correct this habit, she taught me the female piece *Kurokami* which requires the dancer to move through a set of very subtle gestures of the hands and head in a slow sustained tempo. This tempo is maintained by the dancer as she keeps her torso erect and the knees bent at a forty-five degree angle. When she started teaching me the dance she mentioned she was teaching it to me to give me strength. I thought this was a peculiar statement as I had been lifting weights for years and considered myself to be 'strong.' In many hours of repeating the dance, I realized that I was not gaining actual physical strength but my ability to organize my muscles with subtle sustained precision was increasing. As I became able to complete this particular style of movement with a greater degree of refinement, I observed that my capacity for concentrated focus on the individual moment of movement also increased. My tendency to speed through one movement to another and only partly utilizing my musculature was being replaced by an attention to the kinesthetic detail of each moment of movement. I was gaining strength but not brute strength of weight lifting. It was the more subtle strength associated with concentration, focus, and increased somatic awareness. This change of kinesthetic knowledge was not limited to the studio but began to carry over to other areas of my life as well. My typical pattern when doing any domestic chore was to do it as quickly as possible without much thought as to what I was actually doing. Suddenly each time I performed a task, I was aware of how I was incorporating myself in the task. I was cutting onions and becoming aware of how I was cutting onions. Possibly if I had gained this awareness earlier in life, I might not have needed numerous stitches in my left hand.

Kanriye Fujima's desire as a teacher is to help students find new ways of interacting with their enviornment through changing their physical approach to their reality. This is a concept that is central to zen based training forms which contend that the mental approach to life can be altered by changing the physical approach. A simple expression of this is the calming of the mind associated with the quietness of the physical state of meditation. More complex psychotherapies referred to in chapter one, such as the entire field of bioenergetics, have developed therapies designed around mental states and their physical relationship. The primary assumption of the somatic therapies of Alexander and Feldenkrais is that altering patterns of individual self-use will change the individual's action in their environment.[5]

The somatic training approach of the lessons trains individuals in a variety of attributes. (see Chart 5-A) Physical and verbal silence is an important aspect of each lesson. The students watch others waiting silently for the completion of a lesson and are expected to wait silently themselves. Students who do not adhere to the expected behavior are not directly corrected but are subtly guided within the lesson itself. During a lesson when one young student was 'clowning around,' Sensei said nothing but had the student repeat the movement again and again until the excess energy had dissipated. At this point the student began to learn the movement. Students also practice physical silence in each and every dance through learning to comfortably hold a pose without unnecessary muscular tension.

The students have an expanded level of kinesthetic intelligence from their practice of dance pieces that incorporate idealized masculine and feminine movement styles. In Laban effort-shape terms, their musculatures have experienced the strong, direct spatially outward focused movements of the male characters. And, they have experienced the light, indirect, spatially inward focused movements of the female characters.[6] Their training in both forms of movement allows them to change from male to female characters in the time space of a dance piece. In some dance stories it is not uncommon for a male movement phrase to be immediately followed by a female movement phrase. From an eastern perspective, this could be considered as a balance of *yang* (masculine) and *yin* (feminine) energies.

Beyond this, the manipulation of props in many of the dances have taught the students a level of hand eye coordination in relationship to the body. As the student learns to manipulate props of different sizes from umbrellas to silk cloths, she is also learning subtle small muscle control. To be successful at the manipulation of the props, it is necessary for the student to release any muscles that are not directly involved. The result is the student's enhanced ability to complete tasks requiring attention to detail without unnecessary body tension. The attention to detail that is a part of learning to maneuver the props is also practiced in putting on and care of the practice attire. The student, of any age, is never allowed to participate in a lesson in a state of disarray. If the student for whatever reason is unable to correctly put the practice garments on, Sensei or one of the *natori* help her. After the lesson, the student is expected to carefully fold and put away the practice attire.

The studio is the arena for the system of study which helps to develop the psychophysical skills that Kanriye Fujima refers to as 'personality with gracefulness.' The culmination of the years of lessons, the primary component is a greater level of awareness of subtextual information. This is taught through lessons that require that they utilize all their sensory potential during all phases of the lesson. It is also taught through participating in a group in which communication between the principal role models is primarily nonverbal. The primary attributes associated with Sensei's personal goal for each student are: concentration, focus, attention to the moment, attention to detail, physical and verbal silence, kinesthetic awareness, acceptance of position in society, playfulness, and duty.

The personal qualities Sensei stresses have a visual impact that is related to Japanese arts in general. The importance of *ma*, the silence from which the harmonious flow of the universe is derived, is taught as a part of each piece. The student is taught the concept of *ma* and its associated concept *utsuri* (transitions between the moment), not through discussion, but through constant imitation of Sensei's movement. The speed at which the phrases are taught requires that the student duplicate the picture that Sensei is enacting in front of her. This method

Chart 5-A

QUALITIES OF PERSONALITY WITH GRACEFULNESS

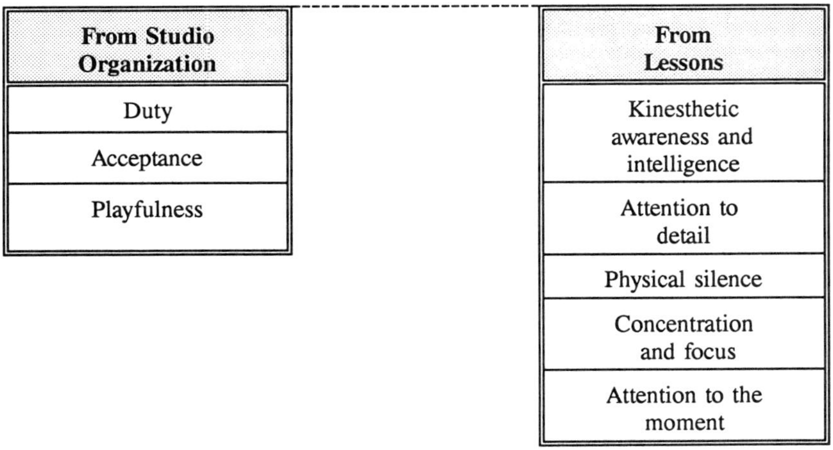

From Studio Organization	From Lessons
Duty	Kinesthetic awareness and intelligence
Acceptance	Attention to detail
Playfulness	Physical silence
	Concentration and focus
	Attention to the moment

Dashed line represents interaction between the organization and the lessons.

of teaching forces the student to become aware of the total body and not just an individual part or a part in relationship to another part. The student, in imitating Sensei, is learning kinesthetically not only how to move from one pose to another but through the transition from one pose to another. This transition often incorporates a moment of physical silence but without any loss of physical energy. As the student memorizes the movement as a set of pictures, she becomes aware of the pose and the potential movement into the next *kata* before the movement has actually begun.

The typical person who studies with Sensei from childhood through her teenage years will never be able to verbalize the concept of *ma*. After all, the concept has never been discussed as part of a lesson. The student will not say that a dancer is able to physicalize the concept of *ma*. She will tell you when watching a performer who does not have it that the performer looks "ungraceful," "unformed," "awkward," or "halting." A person who has developed a sense of *ma* is "smooth," "fluid," and "formed" and according to Sensei able to move with "conscious grace."

Although she encourages talented students to study to become *natori* Kanriye Fujima's goal in teaching does not appear to be to train professional performers. It is instead to teach the students, through their study of *nihon buyo,* a set of attitudes and behaviors related to her understanding of being a good human being which also means being a good ethnic Japanese. Current students, many of whom today are the progeny of interethnic families, become acquainted with these traits both by the physical discipline of the form and by participating in an environment in which the behavior modes of 'personality with gracefulness' exist in the relationships between Kanriye Fujima and the other members of the school. Through their involvement in classes and performances, the students observe and participate in a group where each member, including Kanriye Fujima and the *natori*, are fulfilling their duty by careful completion of the tasks associated with their assigned role within the group. Kanriye Fujima fulfills her responsibility as master by providing a consistent environment for learning, thoughtful attention to the abilities of each individual student, opportunities to perform their acquired skill, and the necessary costumes, props, and make-up. The *natori* act as her ever ready helpers, bringing tea for the afternoon break, preparing meals, mending costumes, helping to dress students for performances, or serving as stage hands or *koken*. The students observe people working in synchrony with each other without the forms of verbal communication that are part of similar situations in the United States. They demonstrate proper respect for Kanriye Fujima and the traditional form by their regular attendance at lessons and their willingness to follow her guidance in all matters related to their growth as *nihon buyo* students. The ideals of obligation and loyalty, and nonverbal communication may or may not be part of their own enculturation, but within the scope of the school they are able to observe others engaged in these behavioral forms as well as participate in them.

Notes

1. This is based on 1992. Since 1987 the fees have increased from $35 a month to $45.

2. There are some students whose lessons are an hour long. They are generally all adults.

3. This is from the June 1990 recital program of Fujinami-kai.

4. A variation on this dance is *Harusame jishi* (Lion Dancers in the Spring Rain).

5. The Alexander and Feldenkrais approaches to the soma have two primary components: 1) to teach individuals a general use of the self that is based on seeing the self as part of a continuing process of discovery; and 2) to help individuals release over-contracted muscles that are the result of social conditioning and personal habit. Discussions are found in Moshe Feldenkrais, *The Potent Self* (San Francisco:Harper, 1985) and Wilfred Barlow, M.D., *The Alexander Technique* (Vermont:Healing Arts Press, 1990).

6. Laban was a movement theorist who developed both a method of analyzing movement and an approach to expanding the potential movement capabilities of his students. A reference particularly applicable to theatre is Rudolf Laban, *The Mastery of Movement* (Boston:Plays, Inc., 1971).

CHAPTER VI

THE PERFORMANCE ELEMENTS

In 1985, I spent the summer in Kyoto, Japan studying *nihon buyo* with Kansome Fujima under the auspices of the Traditional Theatre Training Program of Japan. For six weeks a group of us studied each day the specific dance piece assigned to us by Kansome Fujima as well as practicing those of our fellow students. Kansome announced on the second day of the lessons that we needed to be certain to work hard as we would be performing our assigned piece at a local theatre at the end of the six week period. I felt this was rushing the learning process as I did not believe that I could learn an entire new movement style in six weeks adequately enough to perform it publicly. I raised an objection, thinking that I as an individual student could decide not to perform if I did not feel prepared. Kansome Fujima turned to me and stated in a voice that indicated she did not expect to discuss it further, "I am certain that you will perform the piece very well." I realized immediately I would be performing *Ayame yukata*.

The performance for the *buyo* student is an extension of the learning process. Each student regardless of age or technical proficiency is expected to be a part of the school's annual or semi-annual presentation. Consequently, a program may include students of various ages and abilities from five to sixty and from amateur to professional.

The public performance of the piece chosen for you by your teacher has two separate but interrelated functions. First, it provides another set of circumstances with distinctive concerns related to public performance. A successful performance requires that you have not only learned the movement phrases of the dance piece, but can maintain your concentration, focus, and allow the character of the piece to move through you despite potential performance anxieties. The second aspect of the public presentation is the relationship with the audience. The public recital is an opportunity for the audience to participate as observers in your growth and development in the form. Since many members of the audience are previous students, the performance becomes an opportunity for them to re-experience their own learning process by watching others perform the same or similar pieces.

Costume, Make-up, and Music

Nihon buyo in Japan is similar to its predecessor *kabuki* in attempting to create a stage environment which incorporates costume, music, and movement to achieve a unity of visual and auditory images in arresting combinations of color, sound, and movement. Within the limits of a budget, which is dependent upon community funding sources, Kanriye Fujima makes a conscious effort to create a similarly aesthetically arranged spectacle. To the extent this is financially possible, the formal recitals share many of the production values of Japanese recitals. However, there are many stage conventions found in *kabuki* and associated *nihon buyo* recitals in Japan such as the use of the *hanamichi* that are not found in Pacific Northwest performances.[1]

The stage of a *nihon buyo* performance varies depending upon the event. The dance schools in all three communities perform as part of formal performances associated with the school but they also perform at a variety of community events both internal and external to the Japanese American community (see Chapter 7). Regardless of the event and the stage associated with it, the separate schools produce carefully costumed programs incorporating the classical, modern, and folk movement styles. Each dancer is costumed in the appropriate undergarments, the relevant outer garments, footwear, the correct make-up, and wig or hair arrangement as well as the necessary props for each dance piece.

For any performance, but especially for recitals, the outward visual appearance of the individual student is transformed, with the help of Kanriye Fujima and her assistants, from a student to a character from the Japanese theatre. Although the student will have worn practice wear during all her lessons, it is not until the actual performance that she takes on the entire physical manifestation. The adjustment for the student is considerable as the actual costume can often differ in size, shape, and weight from the practice wear. This can be particularly true for the *kabuki* originated pieces that purposely exaggerate the physicality of the character. The final costume can weigh as much as thirty pounds and include an ornate wig which by itself may weigh several pounds. The student is confronted not only with the anxiety that surrounds any performance, but also with adapting to elements of costuming that were not part of the studio portion of the rehearsal process. Despite the fact that they have to wait patiently for long periods in their costumes before going on stage, the younger students aged 5 to 8 embrace the experience with obvious enjoyment of the constant attention they receive from their attendant parents. The older the student the greater is the performance anxiety. For those who have spent years training in the form and have experience in performing a variety of characters in different costumes, the transformation is the final act in the ritual preparation for performance. The process allows them to transform internally as well as externally.

The costumes for the dances are either elaborate costumes representing individual characters or simple ensembles referred to as *su odori*. The character costumes are based on four hundred years of tradition and primarily represent characters created for the *kabuki* stage. They can be divided into three categories; men, women, and people of the community. They are embedded with symbolism indicating the position of the character in the community of the represented time period. This is information known to Kanriye Fujima which she sometimes shares with the student.

The primary costume for all characters is variations on the line and shape of the basic *kimono*. This is particularly true for female characters. The form of the *kimono* will indicate the age and status of the character:

> The woman's *kimono* is one of the unique expressions of Japanese life. It can denote the age and marital status of the wearer, the season of the year, the beginning of a new life, and even death. Youth is represented by the *furisode* (*furi*, swinging or hanging; *sode*, sleeve), the *kimono* with long swinging sleeves worn by unmarried girls and young wives. After marriage, except for young wives, but strictly after childbirth, the sleeves are shortened. The young wear bright hues, especially red, with the various colors of the *kimono* becoming gradually less and less vivid by middle age, only to reach the somber state of gray, yellowish tan, and beige in older age, although all retain the loveliness of some of the world's finest fabrics created on the hand looms of Japan. (Shaver, 1966, p. 113-114)

A garment made without any buttons, zippers, or other connectors the *kimono* is wrapped around the body of the wearer and held in place by a number of tied sashes. Prior to putting on the *kimono*, the student dresses herself in a set of pajama like cotton undergarments. The dressers (usually Miyoko and Barbara) tie a long piece of fabric in the middle of which is a stiff collar that extends around the neck to the front. This is followed by wrapping a towel around the mid-section of the body from underneath the bust to the hips to decrease the appearance of normal curvature. This towel is also held on by a long sash. The last item to be put on is the appropriate *kimono*. The *kimono* will be one of two basic forms: either ankle length or one in which the hem of the *kimono* (*furisode*) follows the wearer like a short train. The last step is to tie the *obi* around the mid-section of the performer. The style of *obi* blends with the character represented by the *kimono*. The more elaborate the *obi* the more extravagant the character represented by the piece. On occasion a floor length coat-like *kimono* called *uchikake* borrowed from medieval Japanese court society will be used for characters representing princesses or high class courtesans.

Costume techniques derived from *kabuki* that are often used are the *henge* (transformation) and *hikinuki* (quick change). These techniques are not considered separate from the dance choreography but are part of the sequence of learning the dance itself. In a *hengemono* piece, the performer quickly alters, with the help of the stage asssistant, the nature of the costume. This can be as simple as taking an arm out of the sleeve of a *kimono* or the difficult change of adjusting the costume by removing the upper level of the *kimono* to reveal the next layer. In this case, the *kimono* is not completely removed but carefully draped over the *obi*. In a piece incorporating a *hikinuki*, the dancer, with the help of a stage assistant, completely changes costume. This is accomplished by wearing several layers of kimonos which have seams that can be easily pulled out by a stage helper. During a dance piece, the dancer performs a set of gestures which require her to remain in one location. Meanwhile, a stage helper (*koken*) will position herself close to the dancer and pull out the threads of the outer *kimono* causing it to fall away and reveal the next layer of *kimono*. This technique, originally created by *onnagata* actors, is used for pieces describing the various emotions of a character. Beyond these two stage conventions, the *koken* will help the dancer by bringing props or removing those that are no longer being used.

A *shosagoto* piece which incorporates a *henge* section is *Fuji musume*. First dramatized by Gempachi Katusi in 1826 (Miyake, 1963), it has been performed in recitals of Fujinami-kai in 1961, 1963, 1968, and 1990. The dance is generally performed as a set of four separate pieces each featuring a different quality of movement as it tells the story of a maiden interpreting the lovely essence of the wisteria blossoms. For the 1990 recital, Kanriye Fujima staged it as a duet for two dancers, June Nishihara and Diane Hinatsu (see Figure 6-A). The dance began with the two dancers posed center stage in front of a large wisteria tree. They were dressed in the typical *kabuki* version for the character of the *geisha* in matching floor length white wisteria patterned *furisode* with longer than usual *obi* (*datari-musubi*) hanging decoratively down the performer's back. Broad brimmed hats covered their black wigs and they carried imitation wisteria branches which they used throughout the first section. The traditional choreography of delicate, intricate steps and manipulations of the wisteria branches which generally faces front had been restaged so that the two dancers mirrored each other's movements. The two other sections were presented as solos featuring first Diane and then June dancing the complicated choreography to the recorded *nagauta* music in front of the wisteria backdrop. Kanriye Fujima acted as *koken* for both dancers removing and rearranging the upper level of the *kimono* to reveal another level conveying a different mood underneath for the final portion of the dance.[2] The two dancers returned for the final section ending the piece with June standing and Diane kneeling with a wisteria branch held behind the back with one arm and draped over the front of their bodies in the traditional pose for which the dance is known.

The costumes for *Fuji musume* were, as are all the costumes for the *shosagoto* pieces, imported from Japan. They were bought by Kanriye Fujima for the use of the students. The students own the numerous undergarments and footwear that are worn under the *kimono*. The rest of the costumes, including the wigs, are owned either by Kanriye Fujima or the school. The students, in this case Diane and June, pay a small rental fee to use the costume as part of a performance. This fee varies with the elaborateness of the costume, but never exceeds $100.

Fugi musume was only one of a number of pieces on the theme of the wisteria flower that have been performed. Others have included *Fuji*, the dance performed by all students studying to pass the certification as a *natori*, and *Fuji murasaka* (Lavender Wisteria), performed at the thirtieth anniversary recital in 1987. The dancer, Diane Hinatsu, illustrated the story of a beautiful cluster of wisteria blossoms swaying under a trellis of wisteria vines while the butterflies played among them.

Male character costumes consist of some form of leggings, often the bulky tied pants referred to as *hakama,* and different forms of a shorter version of the *kimono*. The *hakama* are worn somewhat like a culotte in which you step into the legs and tie it in place around the waist with sashes in the front and back. There are some male roles such as in *Ame no goro* in which the legs are bare. There are other roles, as in the male character in *Oharame* (see Figure 6-E), in which the dancer wears tights. The process of putting on the costume is the same for male as female characters with the exception of potentially less wrap around the midsection of the body. The purpose of the towel wrap in both male and female characters is to create a tube on which the *kimono* can be wrapped. The objective of the technique for female dancers is an attempt to hide the natural bulges that come with having breasts and hips. For male dancers it is to create a greater size to the torso than may exist in real life. Through this initial stage of the costuming, the dancer, whether male or female, is transformed from self to gender neutral other. The actual costume converts the dancer into a character.

The costume for community characters is made up of the same basic pieces as those of the male and female role types. The difference is in the method of exaggeration. The costumes of highly stylized male and female characters are exaggerated idealizations of what are considered to be masculine and feminine qualities. Regardless of variation, the masculine costuming tends to compliment the outward focus of the movement style while the feminine costuming accomplishes the reverse. The costumes of the community characters whether men or women do not have the same elegance of overall design as those characters which are associated with the ruling class. An example are pieces about the lives of traveling entertainers and tradesmen: *Kami uri*, *Yoshiwara suzume*, and *Tamaya*. Barbara Uyesugi and Miyoko Stroup performed *Tamaya* together in the 1987 recital. Barbara danced the role of the Bubble vender and Miyoko the Butterfly vender. Barbara was dressed in gaily decorated male attire carrying a tray and Miyoko in a colorful kimono carrying a group of butterflies hanging from a stick as they enacted the relationship between these two street sellers.

In Japan, *su odori* is considered to be the most difficult costume style in which to perform, as the performer cannot rely on an elaborate costume to create a colorful effect, but must rely entirely on his/her technique.[3] The dancer does not wear a wig and only a minimum amount of make-up. A male performer is dressed in a simple black crested *kimono* worn together with a *hakama*. A female performer wears a simple *kimono* and *obi*. The costumes for either men or women, although not consisting of complex layering of costume, are made of beautiful silk fabric with design elements woven into the fabric that are appropriate for the mood of the dance piece. *Su odori* performances take place in front of a set of Japanese screens decorated in designs that enhance the atmosphere of the dance piece. In the Pacific Northwest, this form of costuming is used for many community event performances and for small scale recitals. The *sanbaso* dances from the classical repertoire are often performed in this costume style, as are many modern pieces. Group folk pieces that end a program are on occasion costumed in this manner.

An example of *su odori* costume style in performance was the presentation of *Kiku no sakae* at the 1989 American College Dance Festival. The two performers (Diane Hinatsu and Barbara Uyesugi), respectively playing the *onna* (female) and the *otoko* (male) characters, were dressed in complimentary *kimonos* and *obi*. The gender difference between the two, besides the standard turned-in or turned-out foot positions, was denoted by the longer length of the hanging portion of the sleeve on the *kimono* along with a larger more ornate *obi* for the female as opposed to short hanging sleeves and simplified *obi* for the male. For large portions of the dance, their movements were similar, differing only slightly in the body line as a result of the differentiation in the female vs. male posture.

The make-up style for each performance reflects both the event and the character portrayed. For community events the make-up is normally an expansion of the everyday mode of the dancer. This is of course the only occasion in which the youngest members of the school wear make-up. The make-up for classical characters in major recitals includes white paint covering the entire face, arms, hands, and back and front of the neck. The eye brows are painted over with white paint, the eyes outlined and the lips painted red. For male characters, some version of the *kumadori* make-up is painted on the face. These are lines drawn on the face from the center outward with specific colors to represent the emotional state of the character.

The final element of the costume is the wig. Kanriye Fujima has boxes of wigs stored in her downstairs studio and in other closets throughout her home. They come in numerous styles and sizes. There are wigs for young women, young men, *samurai*, *geisha*, and older men and women. Prior to a performance, she packs the boxes into her car and takes them to the community in which they are needed. Approximately one week before the performance, each student is fitted for the correct wig. The wig is then stored back in its container to be brought out the night of performance.

Another costume element of some dances is a mask. Masks in Japanese theatre can be traced back to *Gigaku*, a form of theatre imported from China in 612 A.D. Children age eight to ten frequently perform a masked dance entitled *Kaguyahime* (The Shining Princess--see Figure 6-F). The narrative song is based on an old Japanese folk tale of the relationship between an old bamboo cutter and the tiny baby he discovers in a bamboo shoot. The young dancer enacts the story using a mask to portray the old man.

Adult dancers have performed several comic dances which often use masks and generally portray love relationships between boys and girls or men and women. They can be focused on a potential triangle of two men and one woman as in *Mitsumen komori* and *Kagura men*.[4] In 1989 Kanriye Fujima, who very rarely performs, presented a portion of *Mitsumen komori* for the students and faculty from colleges from all over the Pacific Northwest. The audience laughed in appreciation of the exaggerated antics of the one female and two male characters portrayed through a combination of mask and movement. The story began with the female character identified by a papier- mache mask with a glowing white face and bulbous cheeks who moved in the typical female pigeon-toed walk, but with a wider stance which made each movement large and clumsy. A short dance illustrating the plight of indecision on the part of a woman between two men was followed by a quick change of a mask to introduce the macho male. (This quick change was possible because the mask was held in place by a wooden disk situated in the mouth area of the mask which the dancer placed in her teeth.) He was represented by a mask that to an American audience would resemble a rough sailor. With a highly developed turned out stance, he strutted with an awkward gait that mirrored his overblown masculinity. After a series of short danced interchanges between the first two characters, each time with its accompanying change of mask, the final male character was introduced. He was represented by a mask featuring a pulled forward mouth and furrowed brow which made him appear the opposite of the macho male character of the piece. Although he also walked with his feet turned out as most male characters, his walk was more tentative and followed by an inward jerk of the knees which indicated his general emotional state. The interplay between the characters through the masks came to an inconclusive end and Kanriye Fujima removed the female mask for a final pose as performer.

Beyond the use of the mask found in the pieces previously discussed, there is in *buyo* a concept of mask that refers to the entire body. I refer to it as a physical mask. In *buyo* the face, except for rare *kabuki* pieces, remains impassive through the entire performance. The facial expressiveness relied upon by the western actor is replaced with physical expressiveness in which the goal is to communicate the emotional impact of a moment through the gesture in the phrase as it incorporates the entire body.[5] This method of performance requires the performer to be aware of and to project the emotional moment through her entire musculature. On a psychological level, it allows her to mentally embrace the movement phrases associated with the character. This mental and physical release into the physical character moves her away from ego-self development of a character to a continuation of an embodied identity transmitted directly from her teacher to her.

Like much of Asian theatre, *nihon buyo* operates on two levels that are unified into a single presentation. There is the abstract and mimetic movement of the dancer, and the story sung by a chanter accompanied by some form of instrumentation. Each of these separate elements reinforces the other. Although there are brief sections of a *buyo* piece that are not associated with the sung story line, the majority of the dance is an illustration of the story. The accompaniment for a *nihon buyo* performance still uses the instrumentation established during the days of the early *shosagoto* pieces. The music of those dances with classical roots are related to four separate musical styles: *gidayu, nagauta, kiyomoto,* and *tokiwazu*.

The musical tradition has its roots in the earliest phases of the development of Japanese theatre in the blind musicians of the Muromachi period (1392-1568) who accompanied their tales on the *biwa*. Over time the four-stringed snake skin covered *biwa* was converted to a three-stringed cat skin covered (*shamisen*) instrument that used a plectrum in place of a bow. The narrative musicians gained popularity and were referred to as *joruri*. One of the popular songs from this early period, *Kikuzushi*, is part of the repertoire of every school of Japanese dance. Early in the seventeenth century the narrative musical style of Takemoto Gidayu became popular in the Osaka doll theatre. The *kabuki* in competition with the puppet theatre borrowed the musical form referred to as *gidayu bushi*. This form is still influential in dances whose stories are borrowed from the puppet theatre. (Malm, 1978)

Nagauta or long song is a musical style originating in the Kyoto-Osaka area. In the seventeenth century traveling musicians brought the form to Edo (Tokyo) and it became used as theatre music. *Nagauta* musicians perfected their techniques during the late eighteenth century. The *nagauta* ensemble has been the principal music for *kabuki* since that time:

> Irrespective of these various style changes, the *nagauta* ensemble was the basic component of the onstage (*debayashi*) music of the *kabuki* from the early eighteenth century to the present time. This ensemble consists of singers, shamisen, and the stick drum (*taiko*), shoulder hand drum (*ko tsuzumi*), and side hand drum (*o tsuzumi*) of the *noh* plus a flautist who plays

either the noh flute (*nokan*) or a more lyrical bamboo flute (*takebue* or *shinobue*). (Malm, 1978, p. 137)

Famous *nagauta* pieces include dance dramas *Musume dojoji (1753)* and *Sagi musume* (1762). In the nineteenth century new dances--*Genroku odori* (1878) and *Funa benkei* (1885)--based on this musical style were conceived.

Tokiwazu and *kiyomoto* are respectively eighteenth and nineteenth forms of music that are associated with the growth and development of *kabuki*. *Tokiwazu* music is the basis for the dance drama *Seki no to* (1784). *Kiyomoto* dances are *Osome* (1825) and *Tamaya* (1832). Dances that combine musical styles are the *tokiwazu-nagauta* piece *Momiji-gari* (1887) and the *tokiwazu-kiyomoto* dance drama *Onatsu kyoran* (1914). (Gunji, 1970)

In major recitals of *nihon buyo* in Japan, the *shamisen* players and the *joruri* singer usually sit to the right of the stage (from the audience perspective). The number of players will depend upon the musical arrangement for the specific number. If the performance is of a piece adapted from the *noh*, the musicians may sit in the center of the stage in front of the backdrop of a pine tree. The only other sound accompaniment would be the *hyoshigi*, a pair of hardwood pieces approximately ten inches long and two inches square, clapped together by a stage assistant backstage to signal the opening and closing of the curtain as well as the *mie* of a dancer in an *aragoto* piece.

The dances performed by students of Kanriye Fujima encompass the range of musical styles including *nagauta* (*Genroku hana miodori*) and *tokiwazu-kiyomoto* (*Onatsu kyoran*). Rarely, during the history of Kanriye Fujima's teaching in the United States has there been actual vocalist or musicians. Recorded music amplified by the appropriate sound system has been the principal means of accompanying the dancers.[6] However, Kanriye Fujima or one of her assistants has always stood at the side of the stage and punctuated the beginning and ending of specific pieces with the *hyoshigi*.

Prior to performance, the student's primary experience with the character and the character's story is the movement associated with the narrative. As described earlier, during the backstage preparations prior to the performance, she goes through a transformation that removes her from herself and takes her into the character. This transformation is not an extension of the original personality as is generally the case of actors playing roles in realistic theatre:

The *kabuki* actor does not 'create' roles in the manner of the contemporary Western actor; he rather, in his training, gradually disciplines his body in the inherited patterns of expression. The personality of the actor emerges, but only through the medium of the conventional forms which interpose between the personality of the individual and the role. (Ernst, 1974, p. 194)

The character the dancer becomes is not part of her historical present or direct historical past. To attain this new personality the dancer must follow the dictates of the movement and costume. To create the image of the character, the natural outlines of her body are altered through the use of towels. Her face is painted white. She is dressed in a costume and wig she has not worn before. Within the short period of time backstage and without days of rehearsal in costume, she must undergo the necessary mind/body adjustment, transformation, and preparation needed for the performance. This requires a level of inner focus and concentration that allows the performer to stay relaxed despite the demands of the moment. Referred to as *seishin* or inner strength, it is one of the personal qualities that parents in Japan in the early part of the century hoped their daughters would learn. They believed that the attribute learned in dance training would serve them in other areas of their life.

The Performance: The Kinetic Symbol

Sachiyo Ito compares the *kata* of *nihon buyo* to the writing of the Japanese characters in calligraphy. "Japanese dance is hard to break down into steps because it is largely composed of mimetic gestures that have concrete meanings. This is parallel to the fact that Japanese ideographic letter has its own meaning." (Ito, 1979, p. 281) The *kata* of *buyo* function similarly to the Japanese form of writing, *kanji*, in which each character has multiple meanings. The dancer is quite literally a moving symbol as *kanji* is a written symbol. Just as the student learning to read learns the entire symbol, the dancer learning a dance learns the phrase (the symbol) as a single unit or integrated phrase, not as a set of separate movements of body parts which happen to be working together. This method of training (discussed in chapter 5) teaches the dancer a set of psychophysical skills that have inherent value for her. The students through the extended learning process have not only learned a set of somatic skills, but the living embodiment of a cultural past. When they bring this knowledge to the stage they share this knowledge with the audience.

A comparison of the recorded dances and performances suggests that Kanriye Fujima has created a frame of reference for both performer and audience of Japanese life and cultural values. Within the recurring role types, themes, and images among the pieces there are dominant symbols and key scenarios that represent life in Japan. All classical pieces rely on the mythology and history of the Tokugawa era, a period when Japan had closed its doors to outside influence and focused on evolving a culture restricted to ideas that existed within its boundaries. It is also the historic period which corresponds to the development of *kabuki*. The primary characters portrayed of this period are from the 'floating world' of the *geisha* and the 'heroic world' of the *samurai*.

Geisha occupy a specialized position in Japanese society. As entertainers they live in a liminal framework referred to as the 'floating world' in which people, primarily men, enter to relax and forget the problems associated with their public lives. In the twentieth century, because of their knowledge of a variety of Japanese arts, they are seen as artistic specialists. As such, they are experienced in the 'graceful arts' including the ability to wear *kimono*, a skill unknown to many modern Japanese women. Despite this, their lives are often viewed as tragic for as women without families they can never be part of the normal social sphere. Pieces detailing different aspects of a *geisha's* life are enacted by different ages of students. They begin when the students are very young and include portrayals of the many arts associated with the *geisha* as paid entertainers as in *Maisugata* (Portrait of a Dancing Maiden); *Maiko* (Apprentice Geisha); and *Gion kouta* (Ballad of Gion). The story lines of each of these pieces concentrates on the rigors of the training the apprentice *geisha* must undergo in the study of her art.

Samurai are the warrior class of historical Japan. As characters enacted in theatre they represent a way of life in which people knew and accepted their place in the social hierarchy. A set of responsibilities was associated with the position a *samurai* was expected to uphold. The paramount obligation was duty and loyalty to his superiors. *Samurai's* lives have been recreated in *Kokaji* (The Honorable Way of the Sword); *Hie tsuki monogatari* (Ballad of the Defeated Samurai); *Ogi no mato* (The Marksman's Target); *Kojo* (Feudal Castle) and *Byakkotai*. The later is the story of nineteen young warriors who defend their lord's castle in Fukushima but are defeated. The persistent normative value conveyed in all dances associated with these female and male characters is the conception of *giri* or duty--the *geisha's* duty to her art and the *samurai's* to his lord.

Stories, which involve women characters other than *geisha*, describe the many-faceted duties of a woman to her family. Examples are: *Kojo shiragiku* (Girl of Devotion), *Taki no shiraito* (A Taisho Ballad), *Chakkiri bushi* (Women of the Tea Leaves), and *Omokage zakura*. The latter dance commemorates the brave appearance of mothers during World War II as they sent their sons to war. In these stories, the dancer, portraying a woman of Japan, conveys the image of a woman as one filled with hard work and sacrifice for the people she loves or to whom she has a responsibility. Her reward is the respect of her family and the community. A secondary thematic image in all pieces is the contribution of the role of the art forms studied by women in teaching them the discipline necessary to carry out their larger responsibilities.

Borrowing from the stories of *kabuki* and *bunraku*, many classical and modern pieces tell stories of lovers whose lives, unlike the heroes and heroines of European fairy tales, do not live 'happily ever after.' Instead the lovers' lives recurrently end in single or double suicide. *Kai no umekawa* is a variation of a similar story used in the *kabuki* drama *Koibiyaku yamato orai*. Chubei, an employee in a government money exchange office, embezzles money to buy Umegawa, a *geisha*, before she is sold to someone else. This crime is punishable by death, so the two run away to commit suicide. Lovers' suicide is also the subject of *Toribe yama shinjyu* (Lovers' Suicide on Mt. Toribe). The underlying message of the narrative regards the impermanence of even the most tender moments of life.

Goro and Benkei are two popular characters from *kabuki's* loyalty and revenge pieces. Goro and his brother Joro are principle characters in the old Soga revenge story. These characters have become heroes of the *kabuki* theatre and each year, for the first performance of the New Year, a play has been performed which features these as the central characters. *Ame no goro* and *Goro tokimune* are two dance pieces in which the dancers enact episodes from the mythology surrounding Goro, the most colorful of the two brothers. Benkei, the hero of the *kabuki* play *Kanjincho*, an 1840 adaptation of the *noh* play, is the main character in the dance piece *Gojoobashi* performed in Portland in 1961.

The piece relates the story of the first meeting of Benkei and his lord, Yoshitsune. Benkei, a giant warrior-priest, is collecting 1000 swords as his contribution to a temple. He has taken 999 swords by force, and the thousandth belongs to Ushiwaka Maru, a boy of twelve. Thinking him an easy conquest Benkei challenges him on the Gojoobashi bridge. A struggle follows and the boy overcomes the priest. The priest surrenders meekly and promises to become a faithful follower of Ushiwaka Maru, who is actually Lord Yoshitsune.

In some modern pieces, the dancer may be telling the story of a traveler separated from his loved ones. This narrative line is a variation of the dances of young students in the many pieces that feature a baby sitter far removed from her family as discussed in Chapter 5. In *Chanchiki okesa*, a traveler stops to enjoy a cup of rice wine (sake). The sake reminds him of home, his family, and his former sweetheart, and he becomes sad and lonely. *Oiwake gasa*, *Hana no orizuru gasa*, and *Hana to ryuu* are all about men of fortune who go where chance takes them and have no permanent home. They can never fall in love and establish the relationships that go with having a family.

The focus of some dances is to tell a story through one or more abstract images of the natural beauty of Japan. These dances use an overlapping series of images to illustrate several aspects of Japan in one dance. For instance, *Kasabutai*, a dance in two parts, describes the qualities of Japanese cuisine in the growth of the bamboo shoot, a staple of Japanese dining, as well as the seasonal varieties associated with its growth. *Aki no irokusa*, a dance from the *kabuki* theatre, combines a portrayal of life of women in the employ of a princess with the beauty of the autumn flowers. *Ayame yukata* celebrates the famous *kabuki* actor Ayame with a dance celebrating summer and the iris flowers. *Koi no umegawa* (The Passion of Umegawa) tells the story of Umegawa's love as a theme for the representation of winter.

Japanese communities and shrines are the theme of many pieces. *Amagai goe* recreates the beauty of the Amagai area south of Tokyo. *Reiho fuji* tells of the beautiful symmetry of cone-shaped Mount Fuji. The beauty of the mountain is represented in a series of *kata* that describe its snow-covered starkness in the winter to classic splendor against the blue sky of summer. These and other dances describe, in the songs and the movements of the dancers, the variety of places and scenes that make up Japan.

In the majority of the dances, whether they focus on history, women's role in society, the seasons, or a specific locale, the basic theme is intermixed with images from nature. One of these consistent images, already mentioned, is the symbol of imperial power, the chrysanthemum. Another is the pine tree, a feature of several dances, including *Matsu zukushi* (Many Shapes of the Pine Tree) and *Seki no go hon machi*. *Matsu zukushi* illustrates, with the use of fans, different kinds of pine trees: the graceful pine tree by the pond, a misshapen pine tree on a cliff, and a lone pine tree in a rock garden. *Seki no go hon machi* celebrates the strength and endurance of the pine tree in the story of five pine trees planted next to the ocean by a prehistoric deity. A lord wants to cut them down because of their uneven number, but in the end he does not.

Flowers in general are an image around which many stories are built. There are several dances whose names incorporate *hana*, the word for flower. The dancers fold and unfold fans in *Chiyo gami no hana* to represent flowers of different shapes during different seasons of the year--delicate peach blossoms for the peach festival, pear blossoms for the August moon celebration, and shiny gold and silver flowers for New Year's. The wisteria flower not only represents the Fujima school, but the gracefulness of women. This theme is further portrayed in a piece called *Hana* in which women enact the art of flower arranging. In the process of arranging the flowers, the dancers place each flower in its correct place and are reminded of the beauty of their own lives.

Birds are also central metaphors in several pieces. *Hoo no mai* uses the mystical phoenix to evoke the strength and elegance of nature in general. *Yuname chidori* compares a quiet evening to the sad cries of a plover on the beach. In *Okesa chidori*, a *geisha* watches the sandpipers flit along the beach while she sentimentally remembers her lover. Nature in various forms often reminds women of their former lovers. The dancer in *Ame no bojo* watches the rain and is reminded of a lover who has since left her.

Some dances in the repertoire present images obviously associated with contemporary life. *Osho* (The Champion Chess Player), *Judo ichi dai* (The true Spirit of Judo), and *Yakkuken* (A dance in honor of baseball) are all infrequently performed pieces that fall into this category.

The dancers, who portray these images, have been transformed during their training to what dance anthropologist Anya Peterson Royce refers to as lived symbols. (Royce, 1977) They are not observing a symbol but through the kinetic movement of the performance they are the symbol. As they move from pose to pose in exaggerated physical characterizations they not only portray the character-story-image but the archetypes-key scenarios-symbols that are representative of Japanese cultural history. The pieces require the student to manipulate a variety of different kinds of props from the life of historical Japan from *kimono* and fan to umbrella and spear. The students' learning is not restricted to a specific gender identification as they perform both male and female roles in a combination of styles. Dancers learn elements of the tea ceremony along with the work gestures of boatmen and lumberjacks. There are characters from the historical Tokugawa period, as in *samurai* and *geisha*, and there are characters from modern Japan, as in baseball players. The American student learns the physicalization of these real and fictional characters in the mixture of mimed and abstract movement that constitutes the movement phrases known as *kata*. They also encounter the ethos of the people within the costume style of that period. Therefore, the students' experience of Japanese cultural history takes place on both kinesthetic and intellectual levels. On a kinesthetic level, they physically transform themselves in the presentation of the narratives from Americans to Japanese. On an intellectual level, they absorb the themes and images that are a part of Japanese cultural history.

The attributes of personality with gracefulness are not limited to the psychophysical skills learned in the studio. The dancer in the backstage preparation for performance and in the actual experience of performance is immersed in a set of experiences which re-enforces the skills learned in the studio and encourages deeper levels of commitment to them through the shared public performance. The dancer is given the opportunity to cultivate internal strength (*seishin*) by being required to perform publicly and to conquer the potential stage fright that is part of any public performance but which can be exaggerated by having the actual costumes added just prior to performance. Kanriye Fujima anticipates the dancer will use her kinesthetic awareness to adjust to the stage space and the other dancers who may be on stage. An aesthetically successful group number is one in which all dancers are moving together in perfect unison. This of course also requires that the dancer pay attention to each moment and the detail of it. The ultimate goal is for the dancer to apply the psychophysical skills so that her full artistic *hana* (flower) blooms and she becomes an embodiment of the mysterious impenetrability of life *(yugen)* through the physical enactment of the character's story. It is presumed that the unification of these elements under the pressure of performance will aid in one's incorporation of them in one's daily life.

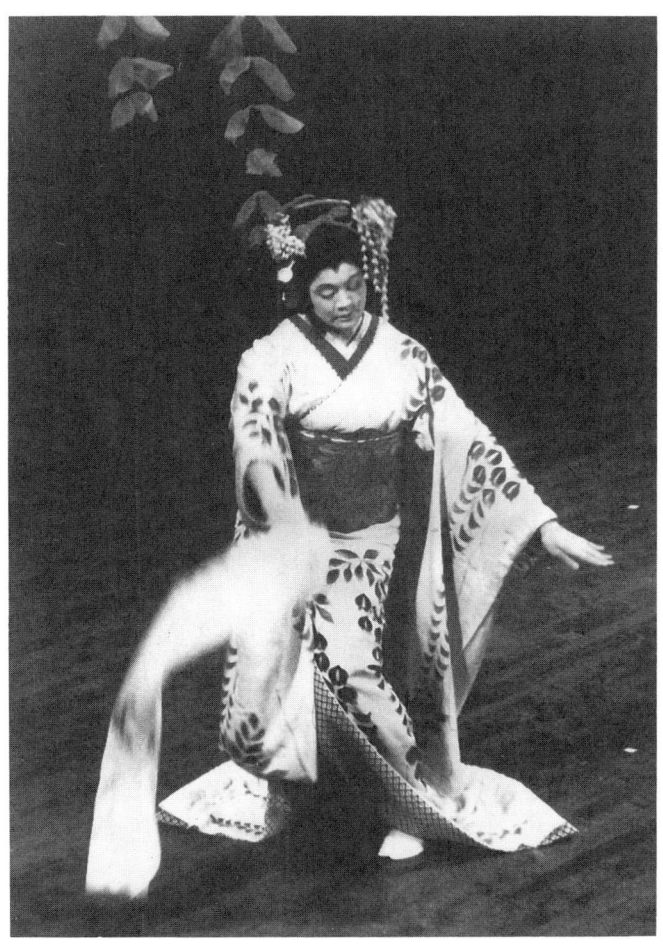

Figure 6-A: Diane Hinatsu in *Fuji musume*
Photo by Terry Tamahara

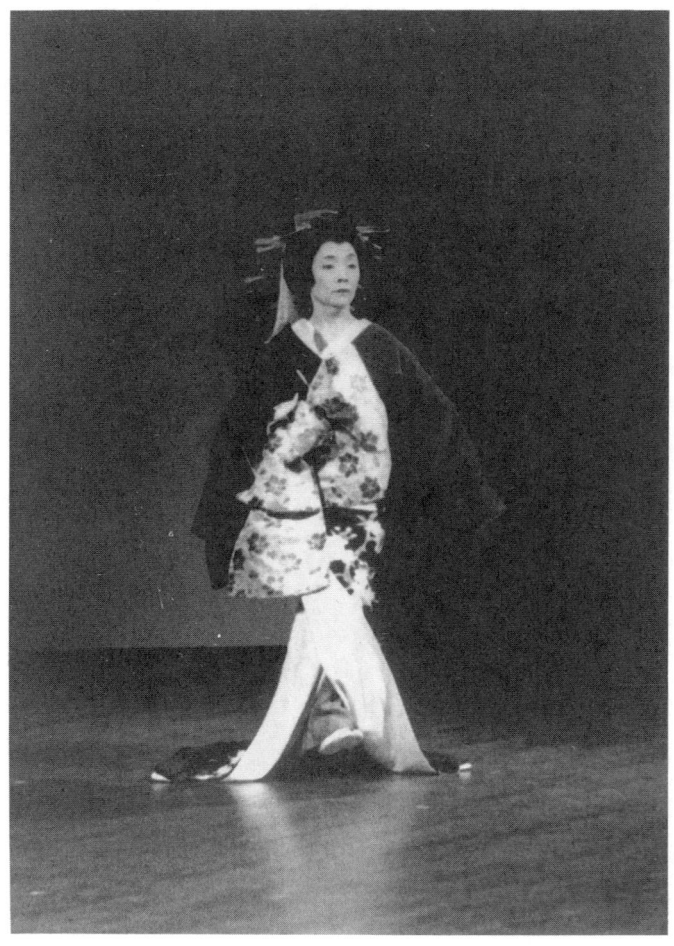

**Figure 6-B: Barbara Uyesugi in *Ukiyo dojoji*
Photo by Terry Tamahara**

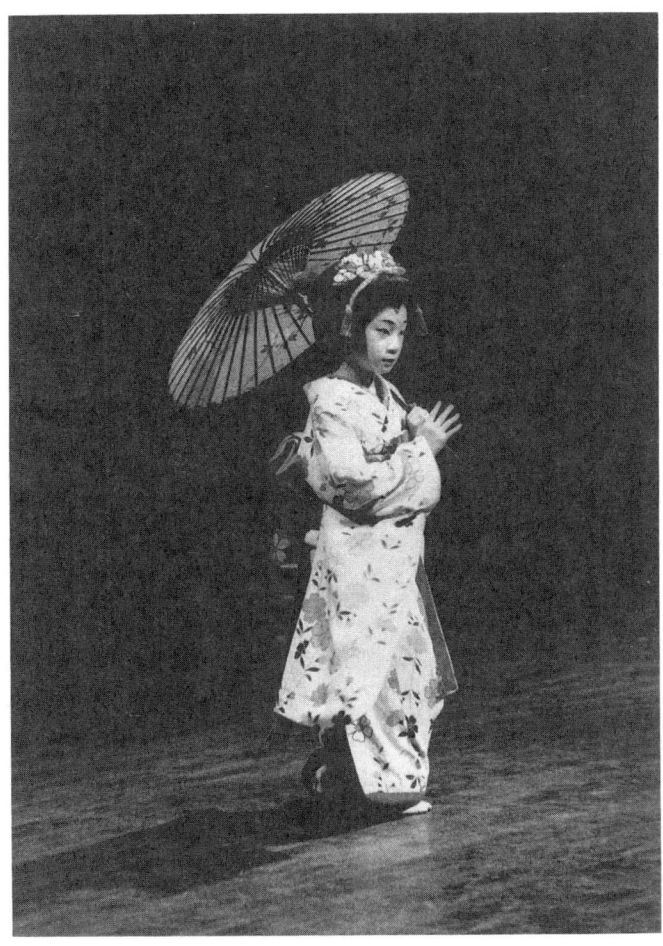

Figure 6-C: Amanda Lau in *Maiko*
Photo by Terry Tamahara

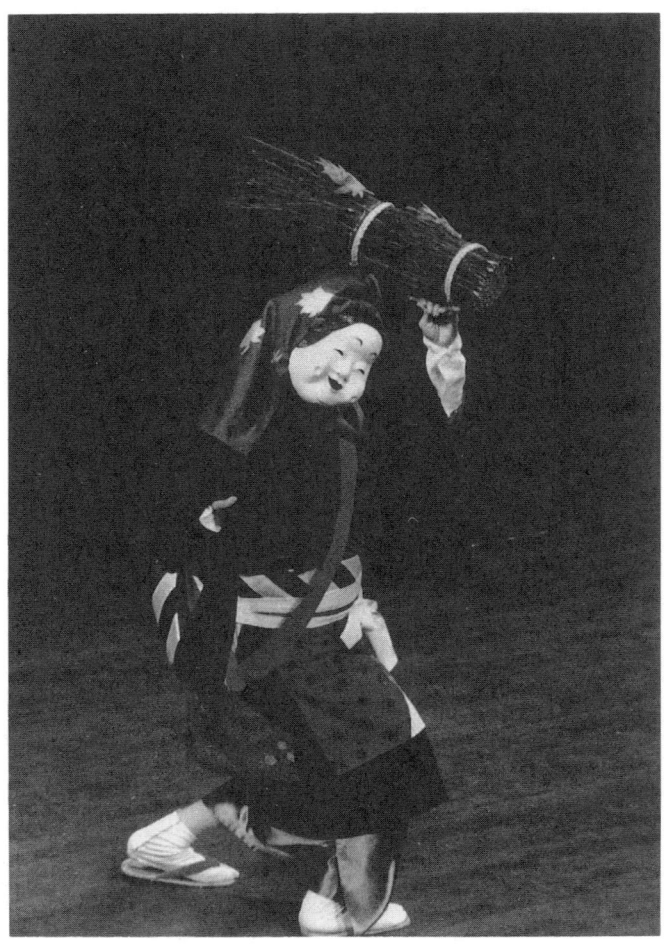

Figure 6-D: Miyoko Stroup in mask portion of *Oharame*
Photo by Terry Tamahara

THE PERFORMANCE ELEMENTS 115

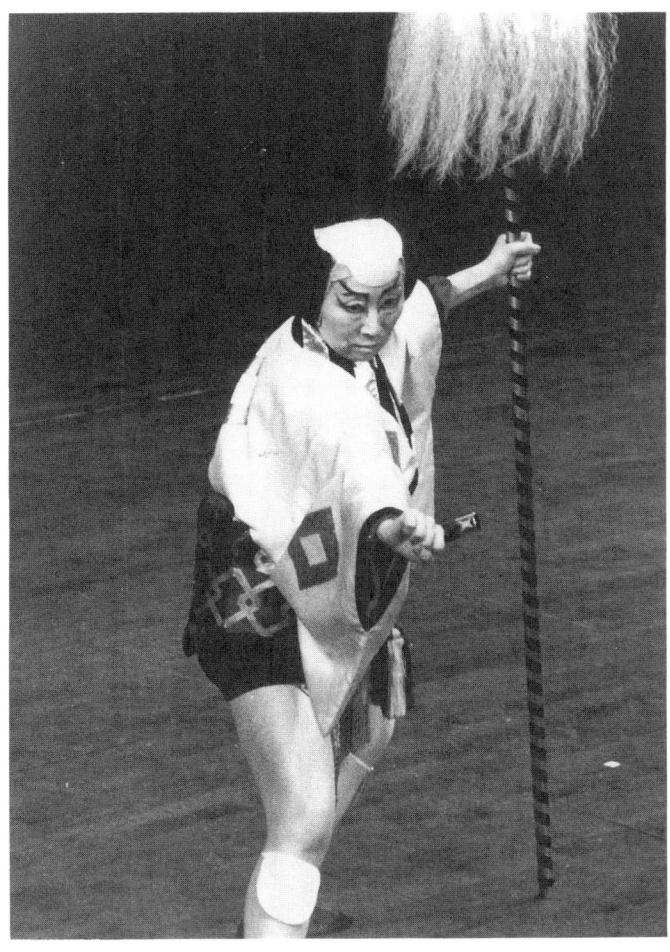

Figure 6-E: Miyoko Stroup in *Oharame*
Photo by Terry Tamahara

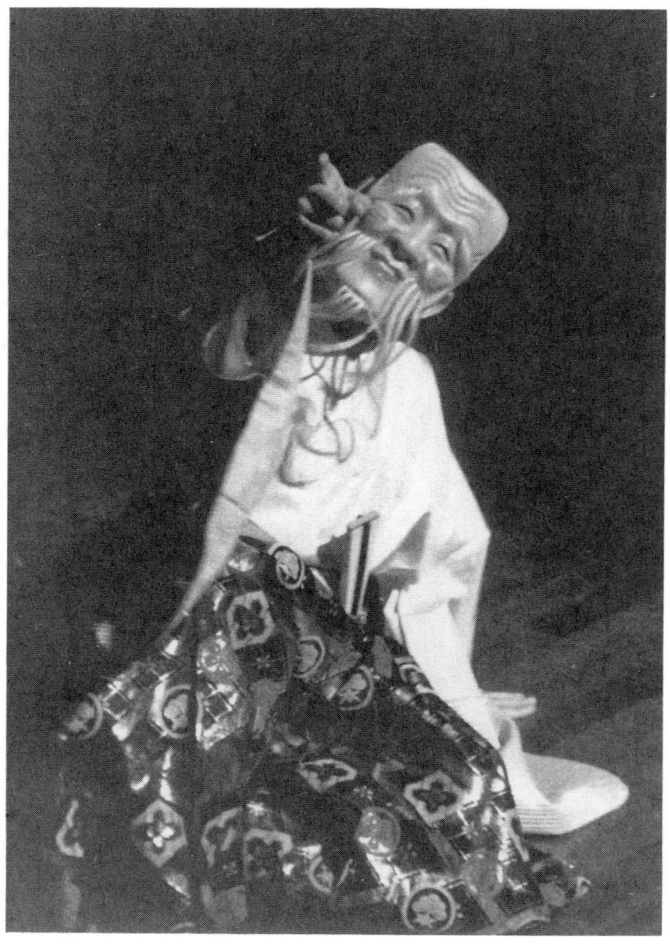

Figure 6-F: Kristina Kora in *Kaguyahime*
Photo by Terry Tamahara

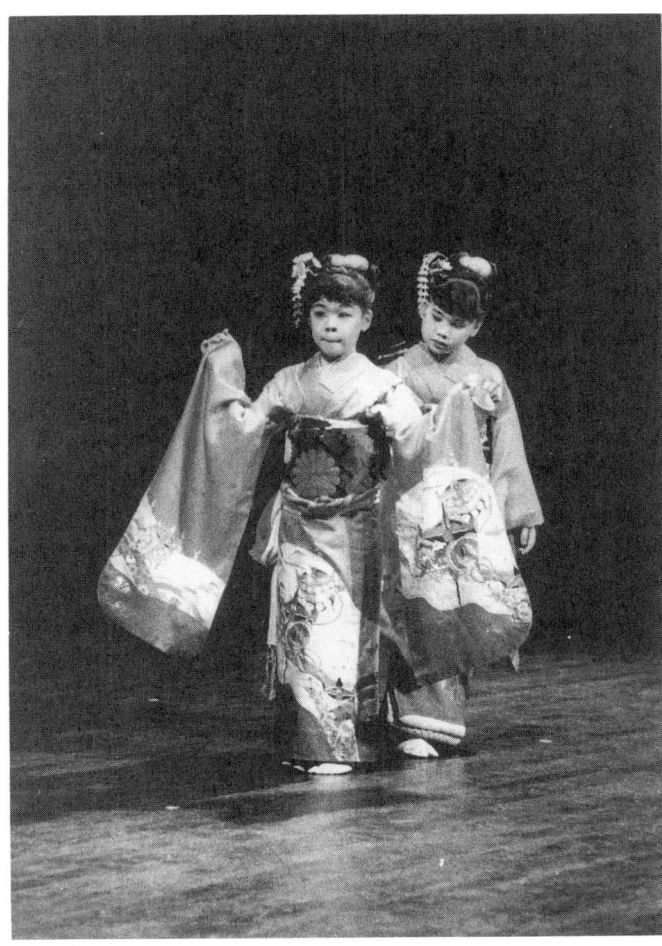

Figure 6-G: Elise Okazaki and Angela Kora in *Ureshii Hinamatsuri*
Photo by Terry Tamahara

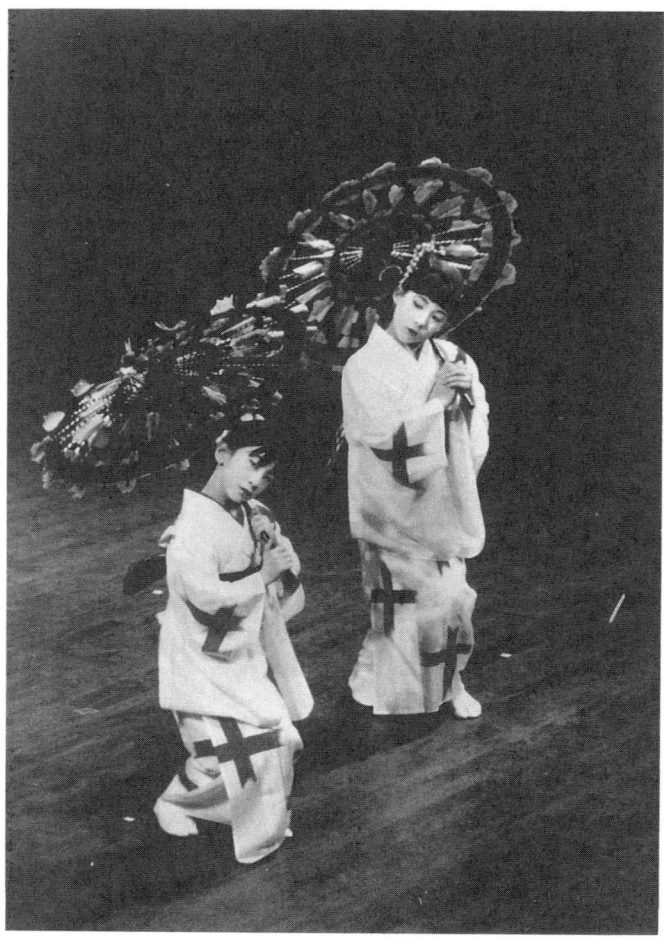

**Figure 6-H: Kristina Kora and Amanda Lau in *Nozaki kouta*
Photo by Terry Tamahara**

Notes

1. The *hanamichi* or 'flower way' is the long narrow stage which runs at a ninety degree angle from the main stage and exits out the back of the house. Many different styles of *nihon buyo* performances can be found in Japan. There are those that are very elaborate which include extensive stage settings, including the use of the *hanamichi*, and those that are performed *su odori* in small performance spaces.

2. Kanriye Fujima places a great deal of importance on the interrelationship between the different layers of the costume. While fitting a costume to a person she will arrange and rearrange each layer to be certain that each costume is a harmonious blend of elements of color and design. In order to appropriately create the proper aesthetic effect each of the individual elements from the bottom to the top layers must compliment one another.

3. There are many occasions in which dancers perform in *su odori* costumes in the Pacific Northwest but the costume does not reflect the choice of the dancer to perform under challenging circumstances; rather, it reflects an accommodation to the movement style of modern and folk pieces.

4. Joyce Rutherford Malm discusses the origin of *Mitsumen komori* in *Satokagura* in The Legacy of Nihon Buyo, *Dance Research Journal* IX, 1977: 12-24.

5. In this mode of performance, the *buyo* performer has something in common with the twentieth century modern dance performers of such techniques as Merce Cunningham.

6. I have also on occasion observed recorded accompaniment at *nihon buyo* performances in Kyoto, Japan.

CHAPTER VII

CONTEXTS OF PERFORMANCE

The programs Kanriye Fujima has directed in the communities of Spokane, Portland, and Ontario, are for both the Japanese American and the non-Japanese American, the most continuing link between these communities and Japanese culture. Her reconstruction of a Japanese theatre form in a variety of performance spaces in each community function to reconfirm a specific heritage for some members of the community and serve as the primary image of Japan for others. By her regular presence in each community she serves as a living cultural link between a Japanese sensibility and the populations of these communities.

The Cycle of Performances

The performance events organized by Kanriye Fujima over the last thirty years have generally been of two basic types: those that are part of another event and those that are held as recitals of the school. Those held as part of another event include performances in non-Japanese American community settings, such as international day celebrations, the local arts festival concerts with other dance groups, the American College Dance Festival or the Governor's Arts Awards. Some performances are associated with specific Japanese American community festivals, such as *Obon* and *Tanabata*. The schedule of performances follows a cycle for each community. The Portland and Spokane groups, because of the larger size of these communities, have been more likely to become involved with performances not necessarily associated with the Japanese American community. In Ontario, the performances will most often be at some Japanese community event. For instance, the *Obon* celebration in Ontario is a focal point for Japanese Americans all over the Northwest.

The school recitals are usually arranged to coincide with specific anniversary dates such as the tenth anniversary year of the establishment of the school. The size and elaborateness of the recital varies with the school. The recitals organized by Portland's Fujinami-kai are generally more embellished than those of the other communities. When these recitals take place, all students who have the status of *natori* travel to the community and help Kanriye Fujima in the backstage preparations as well as performing pieces in the program.

All the performances are videotaped by Kanriye Fujima. Immediately after the performance, she and the other *natori* watch the tape while she makes comments on the strengths and weaknesses of the performances. Until recently, the only videos the students saw were hers. These videos allow the students in Portland and Spokane to study aspects of the dance during the time when Kanriye is not in their communities. Now Kanriye uses the video in the last stages of teaching a dance to point out to the dancer the errors she is making.

Each presentation is directed by Kanriye Fujima, whether it is a formal recital or a community international festival. A *buyo* program constructed by her is a complex interweaving of classical, modern, and folk pieces with themes portrayed by images which stress a number of elements. She adjusts the program depending upon a number of different factors. Her first consideration is what kind of an event it is: a recital, a program for the Governor's Arts Award Banquet, a local celebration. Other questions she considers when composing a program are: Is it a major event that marks some hallmark within the history of the school or the community or is it a smaller recital to give new students an opportunity to perform? Who are the students able to participate in the event? What is their skill level? What dance pieces do they know? Another set of questions revolves around the costuming. Does she, the student, the school or the community have the costumes, including wigs, to support a specific dance piece?

The combined total of the different pieces Kanriye Fujima has taught during her career is by her own words "more than I can remember." The Portland school, Fujinami-kai, keeps a written description of more than 250 dances that Kanriye Fujima has taught (See Appendix A). Also, Kanriye Fujima and each of the *natori* write personalized notes of stick-figure notations for each of the dance pieces.

This notation records the basic poses, the direction of the movement between poses, and the appropriate timing indicated by the verbal cues taken from the lyrics and written in the notation next to the appropriate pose. When trying to remember a difficult dance piece that has not been performed or taught recently, Kanriye Fujima can refer to her notation. Although each dancer develops her own approach to the stick figure notation, it is an adaptation of the system used by *nihon buyo* teachers all over Japan. A teacher from the same Fujima school of *nihon buyo* would be able to read the notation of another teacher from that school. Besides the notated record of each dance, the schools keep numerous copies of past programs and photographs, both amateur and professional, of the performances. These serve as a written and visual record of the history of the dances taught and performed during the time Kanriye Fujima has been teaching.

A comparison of programs from 1957 to 1992 reveals several patterns. First, a specific combination of dances generally makes up a *nihon buyo* program. Second, some dances have been consistently performed since Kanriye Fujima first started teaching. Third, there are dance pieces which are taken directly from the *kabuki* repertoire and others that have been recently choreographed. Each *nihon buyo* recital directed by Kanriye Fujima will include one congratulatory or sanbaso piece and several pieces taken from the classical repertoire that are directly or indirectly associated with *kabuki*. These are sometimes organized into a separate section simply entitled 'classical' or are intermixed with folk and modern pieces around a specific subject. Early programs were divided by the seasons or by a potential trip around Japan. More recent programs divide the dances into two groupings, first, a section of classical pieces, followed by a section of modern and folk dances.

The folk pieces are versions of folk dances performed for ceremonial occasions in different parts of Japan. They include: a fishermen's dance, *Soran bushi* from Hakkaido; *Saitro bushi* and *Kushimoto bushi* boatmen's dances from Miyagi and Wakayama; *Ohara bushi* from Kyushu; *Kiso bushi*, a river-men's dance from Nagano, north of Tokyo; *Hie tsuki bushi* and *Don pan bushi*, harvest dances from the island of Kyushu and the Akita prefecture. A program will end with a folk number danced by all the performers. Since Kanriye Fujima is from the Hiroshima area, as were many of the early Japanese immigrants in the Pacific Northwest, the final piece in a program is usually a dance from that area such as *Hiroshima kiyari ondo* or *Hiroshima ondo*. *Hiroshima ondo* tells the story of Hiroshima and its destruction and rebuilding following the atomic bombing during World War II. The dancers are, according to a program note, "dancing in the spirit of hope and prosperity."

The students of the schools are expected to perform at all school recitals. They are not required to appear at other events such as community international celebrations, Buddhist church functions, and fusionist productions. Usually, a notice is placed in the studio of a need for performers for a particular event and people will volunteer. On some occasions such as the Governor's Arts Awards, Kanriye Fujima will ask specific individuals to perform. In requesting students to perform, Kanriye Fujima seems to make no distinction between those who are Japanese Americans and those who are either from interethnic families or represent other ethnic groups. Her choice seems to be guided by the ability of the dancer to fulfill the needs of a particular event.

The Recital

The decision to put on a recital in any community is initiated by Kanriye Fujima in conjunction with the *natori*. The rest of the members of the school are polled either in person or by letter to determine if they will be able to participate. Since participation often entails more commitment to the production than just insuring their presence, the students and in the case of younger students their parents must decide whether or not they are willing to undertake the project at the time suggested. If there is not a general consensus among the students of a school to prepare for a specific time then the date will be changed to accommodate the majority. Being an astute observer of her students, Kanriye Fujima rarely suggests the date for a recital without being relatively certain that it will be convenient for everyone.

Each performance includes a set of backstage, onstage, and post stage conventions. The backstage preparations for a performance begin in the lessons between Kanriye and each student. It is in these lessons and not in separate rehearsals that they learn the dances they will be performing.[1] Other preparations also begin months in advance. They include the development of funding sources to pay for the concert, building the sets for specific pieces, and securing the appropriate costumes. Much like an artistic director in a theatre company, Kanriye Fujima oversees each segment of this preparation. It is, however, the *natori* who are often responsible for the completion of specific tasks. As in other areas of the working relationship with each other, each *natori* becomes responsible for those areas that years of experience have taught her she is best suited to perform. Barbara Uyesugi has successfully applied for a series of grants and is also adept at dealing with the media. She devotes her time and energy to finding funding sources, putting together the press releases, and compiling the advertisements for the program. Miyoko Stroup is responsible for creating the additional parts for and making the needed alterations in costumes. Depending upon their ability and background, other members of the school and their family members are recruited to help build sets, to do additional sewing on costumes, or to help backstage during the production.

Two weeks prior to a recital Kanriye Fujima arrives in the community in which the performance will take place. During the first week, lessons are given as normally scheduled, but with an emphasis on the pieces the students will be performing. This week requires endless amounts of energy from Kanriye, the *natori*, and other women who volunteer. In addition to the lessons, each student must be fitted into the correct imported Japanese wig and costume. The necessary adjustments to costumes must be made or new costume pieces (such as inner *kimono* worn under the outer layers of costume) stitched by a member of the school. The second week consists of final preparations including moving the sets into the performance space, sometimes a rehearsal in the space[2], and additional costume alterations. Kanriye quietly oversees each section of these preparations. This begins with the student's practice in the actual performance costume during the dress rehearsal to costume and *kabuki* makeup prior to the actual performance.

The actual performance date brings on a flurry of final activity prior to the 8:00 PM curtain as was the case at the thirtieth anniversary recital in 1987 of the Portland-based Fujinami-kai. From 4:00 PM in the afternoon, the dressing room at the Lincoln Performance Hall was a chaotic blend of performers, ranging in age from five to sixty, putting on makeup and costume in preparation for going on stage. The room had been divided up into areas with a section covered by *goza* (reed mats) set aside for dressing performers in their appropriate costumes. Rows of oblong boxes filled with costumes lined the edge of the *goza*. Miyoko, Micki[3], and Barbara, the three *natori* present, first asked the performers to change into the appropriate undergarments and practice *kimono*. All of the members of the school who were performing, from very young to old, myself included, were first dressed in a two-part blouse/skirt undergarment over which was wrapped a layer of towel around the torso. Once appropriately wrapped, everyone's head was covered with a purple cloth which completely hid her hair and served as a base for the wig. As each performer finished the first step, she was sent into the next room to have her make-up put on.

As we moved from one make-up station to another various layers of the makeup was applied by different members of the backstage crew. At the first station, Micki handed us a sticky base and told us to rub it over our entire face and neck, particularly the eyebrows. The sticky quality of the base allowed the white body paint, which was applied by a different helper at the next station, to adhere to the face, neck, and hands. Kanriye was in command of the last station and drew the red and black lines around the eyes and mouth that denote details of character. The make-up completed we returned to the *goza* to have one or more of the *natori* dress us in the final layers of costume.

Although there was a business-like air to the organization of the green room, there was also an atmosphere of festival, with children laughing, giggling, and admiring themselves in their costumes. The older children formed groups to play card games as they waited for their turn to have their makeup and costumes put on or their hair fixed. Teen-agers assumed the role of baby sitters, playing games with some of the younger children. There was an air of camaraderie as mothers chatted with each other, compared notes on the problems of raising children, and tried to keep their children from destroying the effect of a costume. Visitors came in and took pictures of friends, and many brought small gifts, including bouquets of flowers, to the dancers. During all of the controlled confusion, Kanriye and the other women continued to prepare each performer to go on stage.

Just prior to the curtain going up, Kanriye gathered all the dancers together on the stage for the good luck ritual of *Butai Matsuri*. This ritual, which dates back to early Shinto practices, insures good luck for the performance through cleansing the performance space. As the performers stood in a group backstage, Barbara and Miyoko sprinkled the space with salt and then passed around a pottery bowl of full of *sake* for each performer, regardless of age, to take a sip. The quiet accompanying the short ceremony was quickly dissolved as Kanriye began the process of putting the wigs and final touches on each performer. With preparations completed, she proceeded to arrange the performers in the wings for the opening numbers. Barbara and Miyoko left their other responsibilities to don the complex layers of their own colorful costumes.

Each dancer, from the youngest to the oldest, waited in the wings for Sensei to take them to their place of entrance. Once they were situated, she watched the performers from the sidelines, carefully whispering cues to dancers who looked uncertain. For the first half of the concert I took my place backstage with the teen-agers with whom I was performing the classical cherry blossom dance *Genroku hanami odori*. As the four of us waited nervously to go on stage, I tried to lessen our nerves by using the self-reflexive posture I had developed to overcome nerves during other backstage waiting periods. For although it may have been my first *nihon buyo* performance, it was not my first dance performance. I amused my other three stage partners by references to the fact that in the costume and makeup I really looked like I might be Japanese except for the odd shape of my nose, and that I looked sixteen except for the wrinkles around my eyes. Unfortunately, we became too noisy and Barbara finally asked us to be quiet. Somehow despite our nerves we managed, to the delight of Sensei, to stay in sync with each other throughout the piece.

It seemed as if I had just gotten offstage when Micki was whisking me backstage with all the other performers to remove one costume and put on another. In the solo piece almost always assigned to beginning western trained performers, I assumed the role of a young *samurai* for *Kuroda bushi,* the story of a young soldier who loses his lance in battle but, because of his courage, has it returned to him by the enemy. I felt much less an impersonator playing a male Japanese role than a female one, and the turned out foot position of the male character was more natural to my western trained body. Nevertheless, it was comforting to know that Sensei was there in case my body refused to remember what had been so well rehearsed. As I entered the stage my mind strayed as I wondered what the Japanese consulate thought of a European American performing *nihon buyo*. Fortunately, Sensei threw me a life line as she whispered *hidari, hidari* (left) and I began to concentrate on being the *samurai* I was to portray. Suddenly, I heard the sound of the *hyoshigi* (wooden clappers) that Sensei used to signal the end of a piece. The program was nearly over and people were congratulating each other on a job well done as they put on their costumes for the final group number.

The last piece of the recital featured all but the youngest children on stage performing *Hiroshima kiyari ondo* (Hiroshima Folk Dance), a piece Kanriye Fujima had choreographed to a lumbermen's song from Hiroshima. Following a group bow that included the youngest performers and Sensei, the curtains closed for the final time. The excitement and tension of performance over, the entire group, directed by Kanriye and the *natori*, began removing costumes and carefully returning the elaborate *kimono* and *obi* to the pile of oblong boxes. While we waited for our turn at the sink in an attempt to remove the layers of makeup, we congratulated each other on a job well done. We continued to exchange congratulations as we began the numerous trips necessary to pack all the boxes in the waiting cars. To my surprise several mothers of other students took time to compliment me on my performance of *Kuroda bushi*. By 11:30 PM we were all climbing in our cars exhausted by the long hours of preparation, performance, and clean-up.

Although a thirtieth-anniversary recital was a special occasion because it signified the strength and continuity of the school, the same careful attention to technical detail and to the student is part of every performance in which Kanriye Fujima is involved. Her patience and capacity to nurture individually one student after another, which is apparent in the studio, was demonstrated backstage. She situated herself in the wings so that each performer could see her. She literally danced each dance with each dancer, going through the minimal movements she uses during the final phases of teaching the dance. She relied on nonverbal hand cues and short vocalizations such as "Hep" to indicate basic movements and changes in the phrases. Most of all, she provided smiles of encouragement to help keep the student focused. She sensed which students were having a difficult time concentrating, and had varied or even shortened a dance for performance to compensate. She also seemed to know which students, although very competent in the studio, have a tendency to "freeze up" on stage, and made certain that they had enough cues from her to have a successful performance.

On the day following the thirtieth anniversary recital, the members of Fujinami-kai and their families gathered at a local United Methodist Church for a late afternoon potluck. Each member had brought her special Japanese American dish. The table was filled with varieties of *sushi*, rice balls, teriyaki chicken, and rice flour pastry. Fujinami-kai supplied punch and coffee and a celebratory cake. The noise level in the basement of the church rose to a pleasant roar as members and friends discussed the success of the previous evening's performance. It was interesting to observe the ethnic blend: some were of Japanese descent, some European, some of mixed-ethnic heritage. Sensei was dressed for the occasion in a black and white dropped-waist western-style dress that did not at all resemble the traditional *kimono*. After every one had eaten, Barbara Uyesugi presented Sensei with the customary gift, in this instance a beautiful hand-knit black sweater with interlocking gold threads in an abstract pattern. In a voice filled with emotion, Sensei thanked the members of the community in English for their help in the program, complimented them on the quality of their performance and expressed her deep appreciation for their help in sharing *nihon buyo* with the community at large. Her speech was warmly applauded with many people getting up to personally thank her. Gradually, everyone finished their last cup of coffee and said their final good-byes.

Ontario: Obon Festival

Prior to World War II, approximately twenty-five Japanese American farm families lived in the Snake River valley on the Idaho-Oregon border. Farming by irrigation, they raised primarily specialty crops of onions, potatoes, sugar beets, peas, lettuce, and carrots. Although a small group, they established a Japanese American community hall on the outskirts of Ontario. This small community changed significantly after the start of World War II. The area in Oregon and Idaho surrounding the internment camp in Minidoka was classified as a 'free zone,' and Japanese Americans were transported from the relocation centers to help plant and harvest the crops. They were warmly welcomed by the European and Japanese American communities, which were short of people experienced in agriculture. Following the war, some decided to stay in the area, and in time built up their own family farm. In 1992 four percent of Ontario's approximately ten thousand population traced its ancestry to Japan. In Malheur, the county in which Ontario is located, three percent of the population was Japanese American.[4]

The Japanese American influence in Ontario is manifested in a combination of primarily Japanese American institutions that interact with non-Japanese American groups. The social cultural life of the Ontario community revolves around the local community college and numerous local churches. Japanese Americans generally attend either the Idaho-Oregon Buddhist Temple or the United Methodist Church. Those few non-Japanese Americans who attend these churches are usually married to Japanese American members. Both of the churches have annual Fall bazaars featuring Japanese American food and crafts that draw large audiences from the community at large. The community has an *Ichiban* (club) replete with Japanese motifs where Japanese Americans can celebrate special occasions such as weddings, birthdays, and school graduations. There is also an all-Japanese grocery and variety store in the community.

There has been an effort made to establish a national Japanese American Cultural Center and Museum in Ontario. The center would be funded by a combination of reparation funds being paid to Japanese Americans by the federal government for losses suffered during internment and a community building fund. This center, if it is established, will be located on land controlled by the local community college. The center would combine a performance space with a museum of Japanese American contributions to the area and a Japanese garden.

The annual Buddhist *Obon* festival in Ontario each July draws hundreds of guests to this small community from all over Washington, Idaho, and Oregon. The event combines a wide variety of discrete elements from *ikebana* displays to group *odori* dances. *Obon* is one of the primary festivals of many Japanese American communities. It is a Buddhist festival commemorating the legend of the rescue from hell of the mother of Maggallana, one of Buddha's disciples.

> According to an ancient legend one of the Buddha's disciples, Mokuren Songa (Maggallana) by name, saw with his superhuman sight the agony of his mother suffering in the hell of starvation. When this fact was brought to the Buddha's attention, the Blessed One said that the woman, whose life on earth was characterized by greed and selfishness, was now reaping the fruits of her egocentric acts. The Buddha advised Mokuren to offer food to the disciples out of a pure, altruistic heart. When this offering was made, Mokuren's mother was saved; Mokuren and all the disciples clapped their hands and danced for joy.[5]

Based on this legend *Obon* is a time when Buddhists honor their ancestors and the historical responsibility they owe to them. Traditionally, the festival is an opportunity to acknowledge the dead and the Buddhist faith by visiting the temple and participating in festival dances associated with it. The festival has been likened by Ontario resident George Iseri as the Buddhist version of the Christian community's Christmas.[6] A period of national holiday in Japan, it is generally celebrated in mid-July in Ontario. Although referred to in the majority of the local press as *Obon*, the official title is the Japan Nite/Obon Festival and the participants represent various religious beliefs.

The public portion of the *Obon* festival in Ontario is a three-day event. In 1988, *Obon* began on Thursday evening with the first dance practice for the festival held at the Idaho-Oregon Buddhist Temple. Members of the community, mostly women and children with some men watching from the side, gathered in the basement of the church to practice the dances which would be performed on Saturday.

Kanriye Fujima has consistently been responsible for teaching the community the general dances in which everyone can participate and the more specialized theatre dances which are performed midway through the *Obon* program. This evening she made certain that the props for each dance were available and oversaw the music as well as guiding people through the dances. With the drum and tape recorder in the center, the assembled group practiced the six folk dances in the order they would dance them on Saturday evening. Sensei's teaching of the dances was similar to what you would find at her studio except that there were many students learning at the same time. She stood in the middle of the group and went through each piece from beginning to end. She did not explain the movements of the dance to the participants. The expectation seemed to be that they would learn the movements from watching her or other participants. For some of the people, the practice was obviously a repetition of previously acquired knowledge. There were others, primarily young people, who were carefully observing those who seemed to know the movements.

The dances, performed in a counter-clockwise circle, used a variety of props, ranging from a large circular hat used in *Hanagasa ondo*, to small castanets for *Tokyo ondo*, to a fan for *Ondo de bon odori*. One dance, *Hawaii Ondo*, was clearly an adaptation of some basic movements of the Hawaiian hula. The final two dances, *Tokyo ondo* and *Tanko bushi*, were two that are also performed at *Obon* festivals in Hawaii. (Van Zile, 1982) Besides being an opportunity to review the dances, the practice was also a social occasion with visiting among old friends while people munched on the provided cookies and punch.

This Thursday evening practice attended mostly by members of the Japanese American community was followed on Friday evening by a rehearsal of only those performers who would be performing the *nihon buyo* repertoire. Kanriye Fujima also guides this rehearsal which is held on the outdoor festival stage. The dancers are members of the school as well as the local Japanese American male group Tenju-kai. This is a group of male dancers that learn a *samurai* piece to perform specifically for Japanese American events in Ontario. Dressed in their practice attire each soloist and group reviewed their piece, with Sensei making the necessary corrections.

The Saturday *Obon* festival started at 5:00 PM. The Idaho-Oregon Buddhist church was divided into a number of different sections for the various events associated with the festival. The sanctuary was filled with numerous displays of Japanese *Ikebana* arrangements, and a taped lecture on the origin of Buddhism was broadcast from the altar. The rooms adjacent to the sanctuary contained a display of Japanese folk arts and ornamental clothing, such as the traditional bridal costume. The basement had been turned into a massive restaurant with a menu of various dishes from *sunomono* salad to *tempura*.

In the center of the parking lot outside the church, a large performing platform with a *yagura* (musicians' tower associated with *Obon*) next to it, had been built. Kanriye Fujima, on arriving at the church, took the numerous costumes for the evening's performance from her car into the basement of the priest's home next to the church. She and the other *natori* visited with old friends from Ontario and the surrounding area while they looked at the many displays and ate dinner. Following dinner, they gathered the evening performers together and began the task of getting all of them in the appropriate costume. As it was an outdoor performance, the pieces presented were less complicated and only required that the dancers wear basic *kimono* and make-up and not the elaborate costumes of a formal recital. With the help of the *natori,* Kanriye not only put costumes on school members but helped other members of the community who wished to wear some form of Japanese dress. Many young girls came in holding their *yukata* and *obi* with no idea about how to put them on. Sensei guided them through the somewhat complicated process of wrapping the *yukata* around their torsos while tying it with a long piece of fabric and completing the dress with the arrangement of the *obi*.

At approximately 8:00 PM the evening program was ready to begin. Large groups of people had gathered in the bleachers that surrounded the performing platform and the dance space around it. Most were Japanese Americans, but there were many members of the community at large as well. George Iseri, a *Nisei* and active member of the Ontario community, acted as master of ceremonies, a job he had performed for many years. He announced in English each one of the dances, both the *ondo* (folk dances

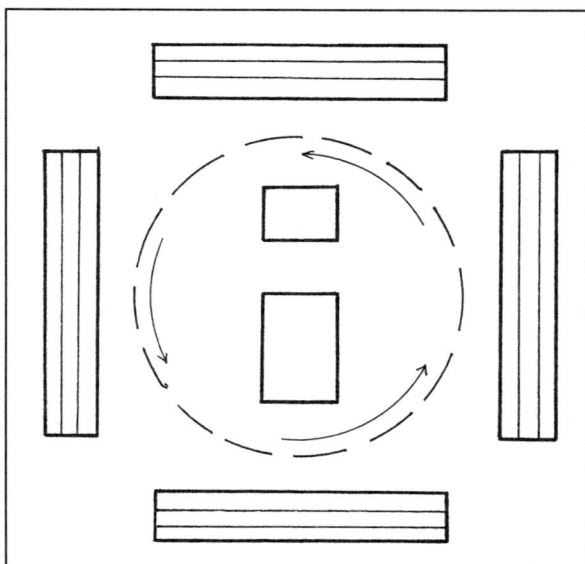

Figure 7-A This is a drawing of the performance space for *Obon*. The stage and the yagura tower are in the center and the bleachers on four sides.

performed by everyone) and the *odori* (classical dances performed by students of Kanriye Fujima), telling a little bit about each one. As Kanriye Fujima passed out flower hats to all those who wanted to participate in the first *ondo* (folk) dance, *Hanagasa ondo*, a group of Japanese Americans, primarily women and children, began to form a circle around the performing area. Once Kanriye had started the music for the first dance, this group of people all manipulating flower hats started to perform the dance much as they had practiced it on Thursday evening. The *natori* and older members of the Ontario school who were familiar with the movement style spaced themselves around the inner edge of the circle so that dancers uncertain of the movement would be able see them.

The formal program began about 8:00 PM and proceeded through the first three *Obon* dances, beginning with *Hanagasa ondo* followed by *Nihon no obon* and *Hawaii ondo*. Periodically, George Iseri encouraged members of the audience to get up and try the various *Obon* dances. Very few people actually did this. The majority of the mixed-ethnic audience seemed content to watch from their bleacher seats while protecting their eyes from the last rays of the warm summer evening sun. The first *Obon* dances were followed by the *nihon buyo* pieces which were performed on the staged area by members of Toei-kai. They began with the smallest children's pieces, *Hanakage* and *Kikuzukushi*, followed by the teens performing *Soran bushi*, the adult women in *Hanafubuki dojoji* and ended with a samurai number *Iroha jingi* by the all male Tenju-kai. These six pieces were followed by three popular *Obon* dances: *Ondo de bon odori*, *Tokyo ondo* and *Tanko bushi*. The last dance, *Tanko bushi* (coal miner's dance) seemed to be the only one that the majority of people in the audience recognized. Many of the Japanese Americans and others, who up to this point had been unwilling, joined the dancing circle.

Kanriye Fujima moved back and forth performing a variety of tasks with purposeful ease through the entire two-hour program. At some points she was leading the *Obon* dances. Later she was coaching the young women in the *yagura* (tower) playing the drums. With the help of the two *natori*, Barbara and Micki, she made certain that all the performers for the *nihon buyo* pieces got on and off stage, the music played on cue, and had made certain that the entire performance was videotaped.

The evening ended with a public thank you by George Iseri to Kanriye Fujima for her help in putting together the program. With the end of the program and the increasing darkness people began to leave the area. Kanriye Fujima was already in the process of removing *kimono* from tired dancers and packing them back in their appropriate boxes. The evening ended for her and the other *natori* at her home watching a videotape of the entire evening and eating *somen*, a special dish of Japanese cold summer rice flour noodles.

Portland: Tanabata and Odori

At the end of World War II many Japanese Americans returned to live in west coast communities, such as Portland and Spokane, which had significant "Japan towns" prior to the war. Much of Portland's Japanese American population lived in a seventeen block area in northwest Portland.[7] Its residents ran a variety of small businesses, including hotels, barbershops, confectioneries, restaurants, judo studios, laundries, and Japanese baths. The current Japanese American population is no longer clustered in one specific area but live throughout the Portland metropolitan area.

The population size and general orientation of each community affects the activities associated with *nihon buyo*. Portland, a port city on the Columbia River, is the most cosmopolitan and arts oriented of the three cities. Its arts and cultural life have been increasingly influenced by its business ties to Japan since the 1960s. In 1961, a five-and-a-half acre site was set aside for the development of a Japanese Garden. Many of the material decorations of the garden were imported from Japan. This includes a five-tiered Pagoda Lantern which was a gift from Portland's Japanese sister city, Sapporo. Within the past ten years, there has been a growing number of exhibits at the Portland Art museum which focus on Japanese arts, and performance events such as the Grand Kabuki, which made its first appearance in Portland in 1990. There has been a steady increase in the number of restaurants featuring Japanese cuisine from the downtown area to the suburbs of Gresham. Portland has an active theatre community which includes a large downtown art complex as well as a civic center for opera and symphony productions. It takes pride in its innovative theatre programs which include a variety of programs with Japanese based themes from Stephen Soundheim's *Pacific Overtures*, to *Butoh* versions of William Butler Yeat's *At the Hawks Well*. Fujinami-kai, the school based in Portland, is the most active of Kanriye Fujima's three schools. With its two practicing *natori*, Barbara Uyesugi and Miyoko Stroup, it is constantly involved in performing for community events from the Young Audience in the Schools to programs with local modern dance companies.

The *Tanabata* (star festival) held in Portland is very different from the *Obon* festival in Ontario. *Tanabata* is based on the legend of two stars, a weaver princess and a herdsman, who are allowed to meet once a year on the banks of the River of Heaven (Milky Way). The festival is always held in the Pavilion of the Japanese Gardens in Portland and is a combination of two events. In one, festival participants write poems and good wishes on small strips of paper which are hung on a wishing tree and sent to Portland's sister city of Sapporo, Japan. In the other, younger members of the community studying the traditional arts, including Japanese drum, *koto*, and *nihon buyo* perform.

Parents and relatives of the performers, people associated with the Japanese Gardens, and other interested members of the community began arriving at the gardens after 6:00PM. They took the opportunity to wander around the several acres of the gardens, to write a poem for the wishing tree, and finally around 7:30 PM to find a seat in the open air pavilion. The program began with several young girls playing *koto* pieces in honor of love and summer. These pieces were followed by the teen-age members of Fujinami-kai performing both classical and modern pieces on the same subject. The short program lasted only an hour. The audience drifted out of the pavilion and either spent more time in the gardens or walked the path down the hill to their cars.

Although the *Tanabata* festival takes place every year, Fujinami-kai does not always perform. Their performance alternates every other year with the Hanayagi school also based in Portland. This is also true of the other groups asked by the committee at the Japanese gardens who arrange the festival. Since it is impossible to have all the schools of the traditional art forms that exist in Portland perform each year, the committee attempts to reflect the diversity of the community by continually changing which groups perform. Some years a *shamisen* group will perform, others a drum group. Nevertheless, the performers are all young people and a *nihon buyo* group is generally asked to participate.

In the last decade Fujinami-kai has been combining its programs with Japanese and American choreographers to put on programs that include the traditional dance forms along with modern interpretations of the same thematic material. One such program was *Odori*, presented September 7, 1988, at the Delores Winningstad Theatre in Portland's performing arts complex. It included choreography by Mariko Takayasu from Tokyo, Japan, and Elizabeth Abts, director of the ABTS American Dance Theatre Company of Portland, as well as traditional classical pieces by Fujinami-kai.

The two-hour program attended by the general Portland community began with *Lines of Kanzashi*, choreographed by Tokyo-based choreographer Mariko Takayasu. It used the lines implicit in the traditional hair ornaments worn by Japanese women to create a piece to express a premonition of the destruction of life. After a brief intermission, three of the adult members of Fujinami-kai,

Barbara Uyesugi, Miyoko Stroup, and Patsy Abe, presented three pieces: *Hoo no mai*, a congratulatory number; *Men odori*, a comic dance with masks that depicts the eternal problem of the love triangle; and *Shishi no rankyoku*, a dance which shows a father lion throwing his son into a ravine to test his strength and courage, and celebrating the son's triumph over his fears. This is one of the few programs Kanriye Fujima was not able to attend. She was in Japan preparing for a major recital by her teacher, Kansho Fujima, in Hiroshima. She had, however, prior to leaving for Japan, arranged the dances they were to perform and the costumes they were to use, and had carefully rehearsed with Barbara and Miyoko how to put on the wigs and make-up.

The final piece on the program was an eight-part balletic rendition of a Japanese ghost story from the central mountains of Japan. Choreographed by Elizabeth Abts, *Yuki Onna* told the story of the snow woman and her relationship with a wood cutter. The ballet was, according to the program, a blend of east and west using as its base the movement vocabulary of ballet and modern dance and combining with it the stylized posture of *nihon buyo*. This program of East/West fusion was something that has become more common for Fujinami-kai. They have in the last three years considered becoming part of a tour to several cities in the Northwest with one of the choreographers from *Odori*, Mariko Takayasu.

Spokane: Sister City

Located in eastern Washington not far from the Idaho border, Spokane is the cultural center for an area that extends into western Idaho and northeastern Oregon. In comparison to Portland, it has a relatively small Japanese American population which is significantly smaller in number than lived in the ten block ethnic community prior to World War II.

The Spokane school, Fujihana-kai, where Kanriye Fujima is no longer teaching on a regular basis, has not been as large nor as active as Fujinami-kai. Over the years it has performed annually at Japan night and other community related events, but has not held as many large recitals as the Portland based group. Recently the school in conjunction with the city government of Spokane has helped to boost ties with Spokane's sister city of Nishinomiya, Japan. In 1985 and again in 1989, the school, with the help of funds from the city, brought from Japan seven *natori* who performed a joint program with Fujihana-kai.

In August of 1989, I traveled to Spokane at Kanriye Fujima's invitation to watch *Kabuki Odori*, a joint production of Fujihana-kai of Spokane, directed by

Kanriye Fujima, and the Fujima school from Spokane's sister city Nishinomiya, Japan, directed by Shikijo Fujima. The program was part of a month-long celebration of Spokane's relationship with its four sister cities in the Soviet Union, China, and West Germany as well as Japan. Titled the "Festival of Four Cultures", it was also part of Washington State's centennial celebration. The *Kabuki Odori* program ended a week which was specifically dedicated to Japan. Events in Japanese traditional arts from calligraphy to *kendo* were demonstrated at the festival park each day.

The program, presented at 2:00 and 8:00 PM on August 11 at the Metropolitan Art Center in central Spokane, was divided into two segments. The first half of the program featured performances by the Spokane school and the second half by the Nishinomiya school. A member of Spokane's Japanese American community, Iku Matsumoto, narrated both sections of the program, explaining the story line and the cultural background underlying each piece. The casually dressed ethnically diverse audience for each program varied from primarily senior citizens in the afternoon to a variety of people of all ages in the evening. The afternoon performance was preceded by a presentation to Bill Burke, the organizer of the festival program, by the wife of the governor of Washington. Burke was congratulated for the general success of the festival of four cultures.

Kiku no sakae, a dance from the congratulatory category, was the first piece presented by the Spokane group. The two performers were Kanriye Fujima and Barbara Uyesugi (Kanhanae Fujima). This was followed by a series of pieces by Kanriye Fujima's students. These were primarily children, some of them of interethnic marriages, between the ages of six and seventeen. Except for the first piece, in which a series of silver screens served as a backdrop, this entire first half was performed before the black background of a drop curtain. The short, three-to-seven minute pieces, quickly followed one another as the young performers entered and exited with the stage curtains open. The dances included: *Hanakage* (In the Shade of the Flowering Cherry) performed by five year old twin sisters; *Taketori monogatari* (Woodcutter's Tale) by a six year old boy; *Tobi ume no fu* (The Essence of Plum Blossoms) by three young teen-age girls; *Suma no yugure* (Evening Scenes of Suma) by two women; *Yuzuru no mai* (Dance of the Cranes at Sunset) by a young man of fourteen; and the final piece *Hanafubuki dojoji* (Shower of Flower Petals in the Temple Gardens) by three teen-aged students from fifteen through seventeen. During the entire performance, anyone in the far left of the auditorium could see Kanriye Fujima standing in the wings following the progress of her young dancers and calling out verbal hints for movement changes. People who were familiar with them would recognize the three *natori*, Barbara, Micki and Miyoko, on stage acting as *koken* for the dancers.

The second half of the program opened with a piece by the teacher of the Nishinomiya school. Using the same silver screens which had been used as a background for *Kiku no sake*, Shikijo Fujima performed *Shizuka*, a classical piece of the love and devotion of Shizua for Yoshitsune, a hero of medieval Japan. This was followed by a series of full-length pieces by five of her students, all of whom were *natori*. These pieces included: *Sukeroku*, performed by Masayuki the only male member; two duets to the celebratory dance piece, *Shita-dashi sanbaso*; and another classical piece, *Hashi-benkei*. After an intermission, the dancers returned for the final dance, choreographed especially for the Spokane performance by Shikijo Fujima, entitled *Genroku*.

Genroku, illustrating various scenes from a cherry blossom viewing party, began as a group piece with five dancers. Shikijo Fujima entered after this brief introductory dance to perform a short *kabuki* style duet with Masayuki. In a series of poses, the dancers imitated the flirting of two young people at a party. This section was followed by short mimed scenes of people enjoying eating and drinking sake as well as looking at the cherry blossoms. While this was taking place on the front section of the stage Shikijo Fujima was in the back with two of the dancers pulling strings out of the outer *kimono* in a *hikinuki* to reveal the other *kimono* underneath. The change brought audible expressions of surprise and appreciation once it was revealed to the audience when the dancers in front moved to either side. After a short dance featuring all six dancers, the dancers returned upstage and picked up scarves wrapped in bundles which they turned and tossed to the delighted audience. This break of the fourth wall was quickly followed by another short dance with all six dancers which ended in a tableau at the rear of the stage in front of the silver screens.

The applause by the audience was extended as the teachers of both the Spokane and the Nishinomiya schools were brought to center stage and presented with bouquets of red roses. The two teachers then led the audience in a traditional hand clapping ceremony of good luck *ichido tejime* (the clapping sequence was a single repeat of the rhythmic pattern 1-2-3, 1-2-3, 1-2-3, 1). After more applause and a standing ovation, the curtain closed.

Nihon Buyo and the Community

One of the primary functions of theatre identified by performance theorist John MacAloon is to reflect the cultural values of the community. Theatre events are, "occasions in which as a culture or society we reflect upon and define ourselves, dramatize our collective myths and history, present ourselves with alternatives, and eventually change in some ways while remaining the same in others" (MacAloon, 1984, p. 1). Theatre can be considered as a continually interactive portion of a construct called culture and shares with ritual the propensity to redefine itself with each performance. Theatre, as a form which must be continually performed to be viable, is constantly influenced by the context in which it exists. This is true even if it is a reconstruction of a theatre piece from a previous era or from other countries or cultural contexts. As Richard Schechner points out in *Between Theatre and Anthropology* (1985) the modern world is replete with reconstructed performances from modern dress productions of Shakespeare and Moliere to tourist performances of native ritual.

MacAloon's assertions on the relationship between theatre and culture were illustrated in the review of the sister city program in the Spokane newspaper, *The Spokesman Review*. The reviewer, Lonna Baldwin, observed that the program was well received by the 450-member audience that was made up of a variety of people from the Spokane Japanese American community and the general the community-at-large. It was interesting to note, however, that she made a point of the difference between dancers from Japan who pursued *nihon buyo* and those from the United States. Although appreciative of the efforts of the Spokane performers, Baldwin seemed to focus primarily on the skill of the Japanese performers. Describing it as if it were a sports event she reported: "Though the entire Spokane contingent performed well, they were no match for the more skilled and dramatic Nishinomiya dancers" (Baldwin, 1989, p. 4).

Her review does point to a distinction between the position of *nihon buyo* in the communities in which Kanriye Fujima teaches and similar communities in Japan. In Japan, *nihon buyo* performances are divided by levels, as are many elements of Japanese art and society. Recitals in Japan range from elaborate productions which include large complicated sets and professional musicians to smaller recitals of the students of any one teacher to recorded music and almost no backdrop. The recitals in Portland, Spokane, and Ontario also vary in degree of complexity but at their most elaborate do not include the sets or accompaniment associated with those in Japan. The difference is related to the number of children who perform in the Northwest performances in comparison to adults in

Table 7-A

TABLE OF PERFORMANCES

RECITALS	*COSTUMES*	*MUSIC/DANCE*	*SPACE*
PORTLAND	Simple to Elaborate	Modern Classical Folk	Proscenium Arch
ONTARIO	Simple	Modern Classical Folk	Informal
SPOKANE	Simple to Elaborate	Modern Classical Folk	Proscenium Arch

RITUAL PERFORMANCES

OBON (Ontario)	Simple	Modern Classical Folk	Arena/Festival Outdoor
NEW YEAR (Ontario)	Simple	Modern Classical	Informal
TANABATA (Portland)	Simple	Modern Classical	Proscenium Arch

FUSION CONCERTS

PORTLAND	Elaborate	Classical	Proscenium Arch

SISTER CITY PROGRAM

SPOKANE	Simple to Elaborate	Modern Classical folk	Proscenium Arch

the Japanese performances. Despite the cost many adults in Japan take *buyo* lessons. It is an indication of status and wealth in Japan for a corporation or individual to support a *nihon buyo* performance. A wealthy businessman considers it an act of status to have a wife who regularly performs in recitals in which the individual cost to him might be as much as $60,000. *Nihon buyo* performances in the Northwest are underwritten, as are most performing groups in the United States, either by the performers themselves or by grants from public and private agencies.

There are other distinctions between a recital in Japan as opposed to its counterpart in the three communities mentioned. Many of the tasks from creating and fitting costumes to building sets and putting on make-up that are fulfilled within the community that supports a school would be done by a specialist in the specific field if this school were in Japan. The school in Japan is tied not to a community but to a school associated with the art form. Although certain schools may be associated with certain areas of Japan such as the Inoue school is with the Osaka-Kyoto area, these schools do not have an affiliation with a minority segment of the population of the community which is trying to establish its identity in relationship to the other ethnic groups within the community. Within each of the communities Kanriye Fujima teaches, the school through its public performances brings together various aspects of Japanese artistic heritage from the music used in the accompaniment of the dances, to the stories and myths enacted by the dancers, to the artful arrangement and design of sets and costumes. As in any theatre event, there are as many people backstage making the performance possible as there are on the stage. Furthermore, the recital in the Pacific Northwest is an indication and celebration of the growth of the child's understanding of her cultural heritage. As narrator Iko Matsumoto said at the end of the first half of the Spokane program, "Let's give a special round of applause to the young performers who are able to learn so much of Japanese culture when they do not even speak the language."

An analysis of the programs developed by Kanriye Fujima in the three communities in the last thirty years reveals that Portland and its associated school Fujinami-kai has been the site of the greatest diversity of programs. The programs in this community have included large recitals featuring works of the *kabuki* repertoire, performances on Japanese holidays and concerts with other Portland performing arts groups. The performances in Ontario have been primarily at special holidays associated with the Buddhist church while those in Spokane have on occasion been linked to the Sister City program. As illustrated in the accompanying chart (Table 7-A) the dance pieces performed and the costuming also vary according to event.

Other variations between the three communities are the rituals associated with the performance and the formal or informal use of space. Each of these elements varies in relationship to the event the performance is associated with and the degree to which the event is associated with the Japanese American community. Those events such as the *Obon* festival or New Year celebration in Ontario and the thirtieth anniversary recital in Portland incorporate a number of ritual activities including blessing the stage, sharing food, and gift exchanges. Other events less attached to the Japanese American community, including the fusion concert in Portland or the Sister City program in Spokane, do not include these activities.

The performance space for events associated with the school varies from the proscenium stages of community performing arts spaces, the arena stage of the *Obon* festival, the thrust stage of the local Japanese American club, the small stage of the Japanese Tea Garden pavilion, and the auditorium of the local school. There is a relationship between the space and the formality of the program. Longer classical pieces, especially those from *kabuki*, which require involved costuming, make-up, and sets are reserved for those performances which will take place on proscenium stages. Shorter pieces often referred to as 'tea dances' and folk derived pieces are performed in less formal settings.

Outside of the recitals which are a part of each community, the performance experience of the student varies depending upon the community. As members of an artistic tradition which is tied to a specific cultural heritage, they interact as performing members of the school in venues in which the form itself is interacting in the community. As a consequence, all students in all communities get the opportunity to adjust their performance for distinct stages and audiences. As suggested in Chapter 6, beyond the shared experience of adjusting their performance, each ethnic group represented in the student population is undergoing a level of self-definition and negotiation of their personal identity in relationship to the community through the performance of the form. For those of Japanese American heritage the performing experience is an opportunity to increase their self-definition as Japanese Americans by sharing through performance their heritage with other community members both Japanese American and otherwise. The act of performance becomes a statement of their ethnic identity. The performance in a variety of contexts is, for the offspring of an interethnic marriage, an opportunity for public acknowledgement of one parent's ancestry. For the student from Japan, it is a unique opportunity to participate in the theatre form from their cultural roots without the cost that would be associated in Japan. For the non-Japanese American student, the performance is a negotiation between two worlds: the world of their personal upbringing and the world of Japanese and Japanese American culture as represented in one of its art forms.

It is important to remember that despite differing ethnic heritages, each student has been trained by Kanriye Fujima. Her goal for all her students has been to help them acquire the traits associated with 'personality with gracefulness,' an attribute of which is to be able to adapt to a variety of situations or, as Kanriye's teacher suggested to her, to allow the environment you are in to be your teacher. Thus, the contexts of performance offer an opportunity for the student to apply the kinesthetic sensitivity she has acquired private lessons in the studio to a variety of environments.

With the help of the *natori* and the communities in which she has taught, Kanriye Fujima has produced a series of programs for over thirty years in a variety of large and small spaces. The programs were at first attended primarily by members of the Japanese American community. Recently there has been a slowly evolving trend, as many Japanese Americans married non-Japanese, for members of the audience to represent both the ethnic diversity and the changing relationship between the Japanese American community and the community at large. She has also served the Japanese American community at large by combining in the same program folk pieces recognized by Japanese Americans whose parents came from Southern Japan with pieces such as *Sho genroku bayashi,* a dance which depicts the prosperity of modern Japan and which reflects the changes that are taking place in Japan today.

Guided by Kanriye Fujima each community uses the *nihon buyo* repertoire and casts it to meet its specific needs. The Sister City program in Spokane, the *Odori* program in Portland, and the *Obon* festival in Ontario demonstrate three separate uses of *nihon buyo*. Performances in Spokane not only take place in the Japanese American community, but are part of the city's program to strengthen its business and professional ties with Japan. Portland, an area with a strong experimental dance theatre community, is interested in combining *nihon buyo* with programs that illustrate an east/west fusion. In Ontario, the home of many *Issei* and *Nisei* following the internment experience of World War II, the dance is part of rituals in honor of the ancestors. Kanriye Fujima participates within each community, teaching, adapting, arranging, and choreographing dances to meet the needs of both students and community.

Notes

1. This is in contrast to western theatre dance training in which the phrases taught in class may or may not be used in a choreography created for performances.

2. For major recitals there has been a trend the last few years to have one rehearsal in at least part of the costume in the space. This means the dancer will get an opportunity to have all parts of the costume on except the wig and make-up.

3. Micki Saruwatari began studying with Kanriye Fujima in Spokane and was one of her first students to become a *natori*. Sometime after that she went with her husband to live in Laguna Beach and stopped studying because she did not have the time to travel into Los Angeles for lessons. After her husband died, she returned to live in Ontario to take lessons from Kanriye. Until recently she has served as the stage hand for the other performers and has overseen the running of a program when Kanriye Fujima could not be in the community to help with a presentation due to conflicting schedules. In September of 1992 she died in Ontario, Oregon.

4. Richard Cockle, Ontario teen choir to perform in Japan, *The Oregonian* (Saturday, August 15, 1992:D3).

5. This is from the *Obon* festival program at the Idaho-Oregon Buddhist temple in Ontario, Oregon, on Saturday, July 16, 1988.

6. Julie Mitchell, Obon: Another Christmas, *Argus Observer* (July 16, 1992:2).

7. This has now become a designated historical site in Portland.

CHAPTER VIII

NIHON BUYO:

FROM JAPAN TO THE PACIFIC NORTHWEST

An examination of the life and work of Kanriye Fujima reveals an interplay between social and aesthetic drama both in Japan and the United States.[1] Her childhood was spent immersed in the oral tradition of the formal *iemoto* system associated with classical dance training. The twentieth century *nihon buyo*, in which she was trained was a continuance of the historical evolution of the interaction between the ritual and aesthetic drama performed by shrine priestess and or *miko* at Shinto festivals (800 AD), traveling female *kusemai* and *asobi* (1200 AD), the founders of *noh*, Kan'ami and Zeami (1500 AD), the Tokugawa period dances of Okuni, the female founder of *kabuki*, the male performers that followed her, including famous *onnagata* and *aragoto* performers such as Ayame and Danjuro I (1600-1700 AD), and the social and political drama of their representative time periods. *Nihon buyo*, as a separate form, was the result of the interaction in the late nineteenth and early twentieth centuries between western concepts introduced following the Meiji Restoration and the established *kabuki* world.

Kanriye's own life in theatre began in a conservative course of study during her early years and teens while studying in the Yamamura school and serving as an *uchi deshi* or student who lives with the master teacher performing household tasks as well as studying. This experience helped to solidify her understanding of the accepted relationship between student and teacher. This early education also created a desire in her to seek greater personal freedom without completely leaving the system. The upheaval of World War II allowed her to participate in all areas identified with *nihon buyo* in ways that would not have been permitted prior to the war. She discovered she enjoyed being responsible for all sections associated with *nihon buyo*, from teaching to choreography, from planning the program to putting on the costumes and make-up. It was a total involvement in the form which she decided would be best fulfilled in the United States. When she decided to move to the United States, she did not remove herself from the *iemoto* system in which she had been trained. Instead, she opted to maintain her involvement in the system's expected student-teacher relationship by making annual trips to Japan to study and to perform with her teacher Kansho Fujima and members of the Fujima School in Hiroshima.[2]

During the thirty-six years Kanriye Fujima has been teaching in the Pacific Northwest, the student population has not remained the same. When she first began teaching she taught primarily Japanese Americans. They were *Issei*, *Shin Issei*, and *Nisei* who were members of a community which was still attempting to recover socially and economically from World War II. Despite the increasing ethnic awareness of the 1960s and 70s, *Sansei* or *Yonsei*, especially women, were more likely to marry people outside of the Japanese American community. A result of which was Kanriye's students began to include more and more children of interethnic families. In the 1980s, there was through out the Pacific Northwest an increased interest in Japanese culture due to the expanded economic influence of Japan. Kanriye's student population reflected that change in the inclusion of more students of non-Japanese American heritage.

Since her arrival in the United States in 1956, Kanriye Fujima has constructed through her schools a training system which incorporates a set of relationships between the aesthetic tradition in which she was trained and social contexts in the United States. (see Chart 8-A) This system consists of several parts all of which are in potential interaction with each other. These distinct but inter-related parts consist of the *iemoto* system, the accompanying somatic training method, the performance techniques, and the contexts of performance. Considered a traditionalist by members of the communities in which she lives, Kanriye Fujima has maintained those elements of the heritage in which she grew up that were suitable to her adopted country and changed others.

CHART 8-A

A FLOW CHART OF THE
RELATIONSHIPS BETWEEN KANRIYE FUJIMA
AND CONTEXTS OF JAPAN AND THE UNITED STATES

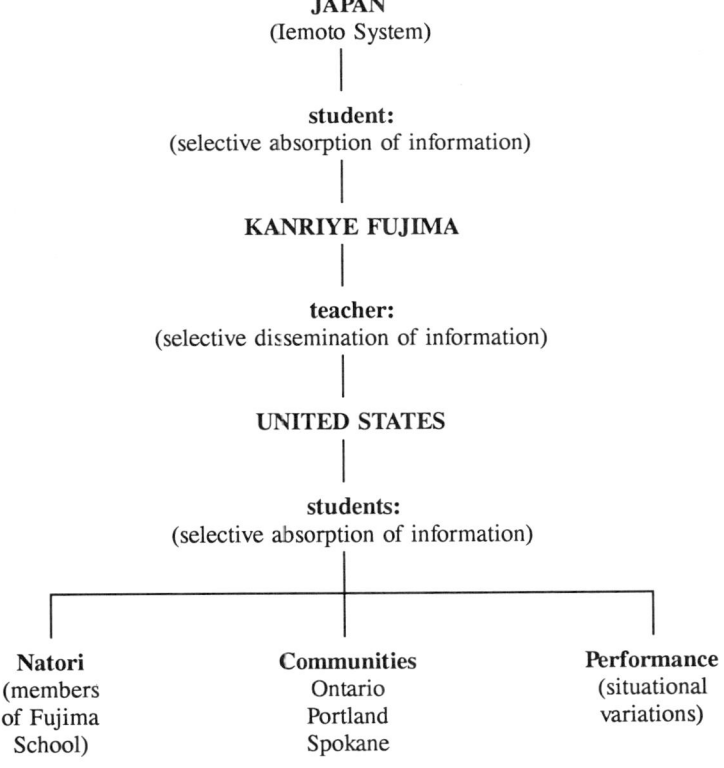

Adaptations of the *Iemoto* System

Kanriye Fujima has since her arrival in the United States selectively incorporated components of the *iemoto* system in the her teaching. One element she has continued is the training of students to the level of technical competence that allows them to travel to Japan and pass the examinations necessary to achieve the status of *natori*. This has instituted another level of relationships between her and the community in the United States. As such, it becomes an extension of the *iemoto* system of Japan. The primary *iemoto* located in Tokyo is the male head of the Fujima style of *kabuki odori*. A major teacher located within the school is Kanriye Fujima's teacher, Kansho Fujima in Hiroshima. Kanriye, her student, has students with *natori* designation who are extensions of the Fujima school in the United States. Until recently, the students who have become *natori* have been *Shin Issei* who have strong memories of growing up in Japan. These women have arranged their lives to live in Japan for several months, studying with Kanriye Fujima's teacher in Hiroshima and paying the $10,000 fee for certification. They are willing to organize their personal lives around the performances of the schools in all three communities.

The organization of schools in Portland and Ontario fit Hsu's description of the hierarchy involved in the *iemoto* system. The *natori* are clearly in a separate category from the other students. The two *natori*, Barbara Uyesugi and Miyoko Stroup, are as devoted to Kanriye Fujima and the continuation of the teaching as she is. Although they each have individual jobs, families, and other responsibilities, they rearrange all of these so they can fulfill their *on* (reciprocal obligation) as students to her and the schools. Barbara describes it as a 'special relationship' of mutual duty. This 'special relationship' exists in the appropriate etiquette while taking lessons, helping with recitals, the interchange of gifts at New Years and rites of passage such as high school graduation, and the household duties that they take upon themselves when they go to Ontario to study with her. They can and do teach students on their own. They assume responsibility for performances when Kanriye Fujima cannot attend.[3] They are the only ones allowed to participate in another student's lesson.

Whether making preparations for a recital or preparing a meal, Kanriye Fujima and the *natori* work in synchrony with each other without the verbal communication that is characteristic of many European American households. Over years of working together, Kanriye Fujima and the *natori* have evolved a pattern of relationship in which each person understands which tasks they do best without a need for discussion. There is a constant awareness of each other and each other's needs. Although not a completely equal relationship, there is a greater perceived degree of shared support between Kanriye Fujima and the *natori* than they believe exists in similar relationships in Japan. Kanriye Fujima does not anticipate that when the *natori* are in residence with her that they will take care of all the preparations for a meal or the cleaning of her home. Kanriye also does not expect to receive large sums of money for teaching or arranging performances such as are associated with schools in Japan. (Havens, 1982) The *natori*, who have experience with teachers in Japan, often discuss how different their relationship with Kanriye Fujima is in comparison to teachers in Japan.

Part of the concept of *on* is both loyalty and trust between teacher and student. It would be considered disloyal for a student of *nihon buyo* either in the United States or Japan to begin study with one Fujima teacher and then go on to study with another Fujima teacher or a teacher from another *nihon buyo* school without special permission from her original teacher. The teacher trusts the student to be loyal, and the student trusts that the teacher will fashion the student's learning in a way that will insure her development as person and artist. Kanriye has an obligation to her students to work patiently with them, encouraging them to grow in all aspects of their artistic and personal lives. Their obligation to her is to be disciplined students who study the form seriously. They manifest their *kansha* or gratefulness through helping to maintain the form through the continued growth and development of the schools associated with it even after they are no longer students. Nevertheless, Kanriye Fujima does not assume, as her teacher in Japan did, that her students will study with her for a lifetime.

A second element she has preserved from the *iemoto* system is the teaching style associated with all the traditional arts in Japan. The primary aspect of this she has transported to the United States is the complete control of the learning and performing process of the students. The relationship first established among *Issei* and *Nisei* students when she started teaching is still accepted by today's students and their parents. The primary organizing relationship is the individual lesson. Other important elements are somatic training through nonverbal communication and teaching the dance pieces as whole body phrases rather than individualized parts. The teaching method allows her to approach an individual student at her ability level. Kanriye can choose those pieces which will help the student grow in the personal qualities she is trying to teach.

Kanriye Fujima's teaching is an extension of the Fujima school and the *iemoto* system in the United States. She has developed a tripartite hierarchy with herself at the top, followed by the natori, and finally the other students. She is the complete master of the students' studies with her, however as mentioned earlier, there are clearly differences between her relationship with her *natori* and similar relationships in Japan. She has adapted the *iemoto* system to an American environment in which the *iemoto* system does not exist outside her schools. The system functions differently for two sets of students: *Shin Issei*, born in Japan, and Americans, Japanese and others born in the United States. For those born in Japan, the schools are a means of duplicating the Japanese experience of a peer group which provides a sense of security within the established authority and continuity of the group. For those born in the United States, the schools are an exploration of a self through an art form. For Japanese Americans and children of interethnic marriages, the exploration of self is also an exploration of ancestral heritage.

Kanriye Fujima's ability to maintain the primary base of the *iemoto* system, the relationship between student and teacher, within a foreign environment indicates the strength and flexibility of a system whose main operating component is the relationship between student and teacher. James Brandon discusses change within the *iemoto* system in an article for *Drama Review*:

> The ideal pupil so completely absorbs the totality of the way, that his approach and his master's are one. Change is not denied in this view, only its importance is. It is assumed that change will take place and that when it occurs it will be incorporated into the broad stream of the actor's way of art, causing no more than a ripple on its surface. (Brandon, 1989, p. 45)

Kanriye Fujima had so thoroughly absorbed the method in which she was trained that despite other strategies of auditory and visual teaching available to her in the United States she has continued the approach in which she had been trained. When change has taken place in her relationship to her students she has not fought it, but accepted it as part of what America had to teach her. The *iemoto* system is often considered a enclosed entity perpetuating a specific tradition. Kanriye Fujima's teaching in the Pacific Northwest indicates that the *iemoto* system with its emphasis on direct individual transmission enables it to respond to changes in its socio-cultural environment.

Chart 8-B

**Qualities of Personality with Gracefulness
acquired from
Different Aspects of Training**

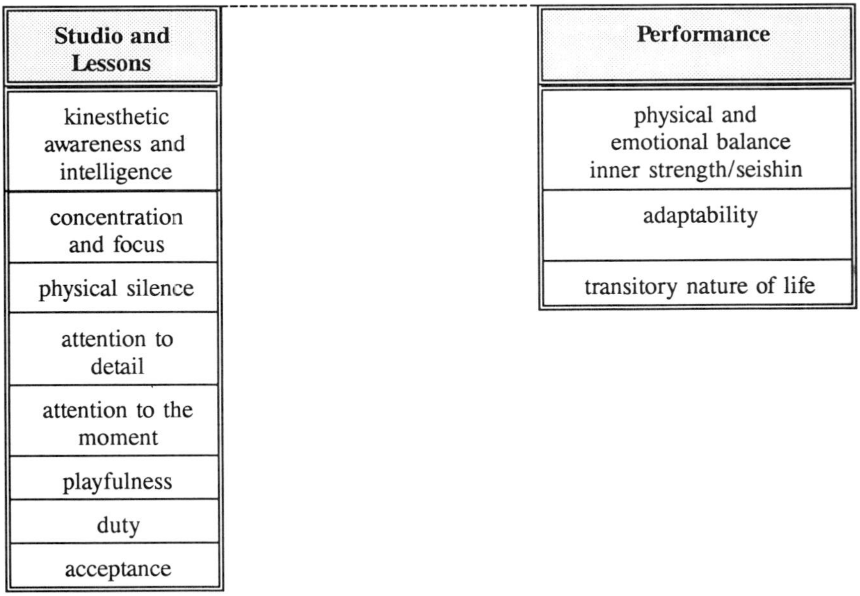

Studio and Lessons	Performance
kinesthetic awareness and intelligence	physical and emotional balance inner strength/seishin
concentration and focus	adaptability
physical silence	transitory nature of life
attention to detail	
attention to the moment	
playfulness	
duty	
acceptance	

Dashed line represents potential re-enforcement of qualities in an individual through participating in both environments over their years of training.

The traditional Japanese interdependency between teacher and student is carried out in the relationship between Kanriye Fujima and her students. She creates a process of learning that consistently helps them to attain their greatest potential as dancers and as people. They repay her patient teaching with love and continuing respect. Although many of them stop taking lessons once they graduate from high school and go on to college, they hope that Sensei will still be teaching when they have children so that their children may have the same experience.

Realization of Training

The goal for the student is not restricted to technical virtuosity but in the self-actualization gained from participating in the atmosphere of the traditional form. In her teaching of Japanese dance theatre Kanriye Fujima helps each student to strengthen those elements of their personality that for her are part of the complex of psychophysical traits she refers to as the 'personality with gracefulness'. The students learn these qualities partly in the studio (see Chart 8-B). There they learn duty, acceptance, playfulness, concentration, focus, physical silence, attention to detail, ability to take in large bodies of sensory information, awareness of the moment, and manipulation of small objects. During performance these qualities are further absorbed into the students psychophysical being. The performance context also promotes another set of qualities--physical and emotional balance (*seishin*), adaptability, and an appreciation for the transitory nature of life. These qualities are not separate from the normative values of Japanese society, but instead, the set of qualities she refers to as 'personality with gracefulness' are the embodiment of the Japanese cultural values of *omoiyari* (empathetic sensitivity), *gaman* (perseverance), and *enryo* (self-restraint). As such they are directly tied to the communicational style of Japanese society.

As Barnlund documents in *Public and Private Self in Japan and the United States* (1975), there is a decided difference in the interactional styles of Japanese and European American population groups. The majority of European American population values direct verbal communication. The importance in these interactions is to spontaneously establish a relationship through a series of self disclosing statements. This communicational style is dissimilar from the non-verbal inter-responsiveness to each other within Japanese community life. As Kitano points out in *Japanese Americans: Evolution of a Subculture* (1976) many of the original Japanese immigrants adapted the codified set of Japanese norms and related interpersonal style to life in the United States. Despite individual and generational differences, Japanese Americans still use a communicational style that relies on nonverbal sensitivity. As Frank Miyamoto observes of second generation, *Nisei*:

> Americans are more spontaneous than the Japanese because they are freer to express their feelings and emotions, are not as restrained by considerations of the feelings of others, and are less concerned about the attitudes of others toward their own person. They are also more spontaneous because their attention is more directed to the subjective self, to (their) own feelings and interests, and they are better prepared to respond independently. The *Nisei,* habituated to focusing on the other, had the wrong habits to build spontaneity. (Miyamoto, 1986, p.38)

O'Brien and Fugita in their 1983 study of Californians with Japanese ancestry discovered that this interactional style still existed in the *Sansei* population:

> In our survey in California what is perhaps most striking is that even among the most assimilated portion of the Japanese American community, the third generation *Sansei*, there is a strong feeling that there remain large differences between Japanese and Caucasian ways of interacting. Slightly more than half (50.9%) of the *Sansei* reported that differences between Japanese and Caucasian ways persist in business. Slightly less than half (46.3%) saw such differences in social situations while 74.4 percent and 65.8 percent reported differences in interpersonal styles in church and family respectively. (O'Brien and Fugita, 1991, p. 109)

Or as Dorine Kondo describes it:

> Culture and meaning, though for many years I had no name for these abstractions, lay in an awareness of assumptions, deeply felt, that shaped everyday life in the Japanese American community where I grew up. Mostly these assumptions had to do with the proper conduct of human relationships: the eloquence of silence, the significance of reciprocity, the need to attend closely to nuance, subtlety, ellipsis. Such deeply held

> orientations, imbued with moral, emotional, and intellectual significance, were sometimes at sharp variance with dominant cultural modes of action, and thus radically cast into relief the socially constituted nature of both 'their' assumptions and 'ours.' (Kondo, 1990, p. 300)

Their ability to pay attention to detail, concentrate on large amounts of nonverbal information, and develop a sense of stillness is encouraged by the method which Kanriye Fujima uses to teach the dance pieces. These skills can contribute to their ability to participate in a high context community which places a high value on a number of abilities related to nonverbal methods of communication and understanding. This increased sensitivity is developed from paying attention to the details of your surrounding environment and extending your conscious awareness into the feeling state of those around you. The Japanese phrase for it is *omoiyari* or empathetic understanding. A related phrase used by early Japanese immigrants to the United States is referred to as *ninjo* or human sensibility.

Omoiyari is, according to anthropologist Takie Sugiyama Lebra, the ability to nonverbally understand the feeling state of another. It dictates that the participant in the communication extend her attention away from self and into the details of another's life. "The ideal in *omoiyari* is for Ego to enter into Alter's *kokoro*, 'heart,' and to absorb all information about Alter's feelings without being told verbally" (Lebra, 1976, p. 38). On a daily level it assumes an attention to the detail of another's life so that their needs can be anticipated without the need for verbal communication. The term for this social effect of this form of interaction is *ninjo*:

> By *ninjo*, the Japanese mean two attitudes without consciously distinguishing between them: (1) indulgence of Ego's natural inclination or desire in disregard of *giri* ("social obligations"), and (2) empathetic understanding and tolerance of Alter's desire which may go against Ego's. "It is *ninjo*," a Japanese would say, "for a man to wish to marry a girl he has chosen." He would also say, "It is *ninjo* to let him have his way." In the world *ninjo*, self-indulgence seems to merge with empathetic consideration for others. The common usage of this term may facilitate social fusion, where one makes no distinction between his own and other's desire. (Lebra, 1976, p. 46)

In social situations this quality is manifested in an individual's anticipation of another's needs. There have been countless times in observing the social interchange of Sensei with students and between the *natori* when they have performed some task in response to a perceived need of another person. Each student, both in the lessons and during the short interchanges before and after each lesson, was responded to individually depending upon their separate personalities and their reaction to the specific lesson. Although the general rule was absolute quiet during lessons, this rule was ignored during the lessons of a very self-conscious student or when a particular student was having a difficult time with one of the dance pieces. During those lessons, the *natori* and others present would talk quietly among themselves as if totally ignoring the lesson. Generally, adult students were expected to put on their own practice attire but when a student arrived emotionally upset either Sensei or one of the *natori* would automatically ask if they could help. The lessons themselves were based on Sensei's perception of the mental state of each student.

Among the students, the *natori* serve as constant embodiment of these values. The position of *natori* is not ascribed as part of being either a student of *nihon buyo* or Japanese American. It is an achieved status given to individual students as an indication of their expertise within the form and by extension their knowledge of Japanese cultural values.

Conversation which is the focus of relationships between most European Americans of my acquaintance, is not the primary means of communication between the *natori*. They visit with each other somewhat during breaks between lessons and after meals, but the rest of their time, whether working at some task or relaxing, is spent largely in silence. They seem content to be aware of each other's presence without feeling the need for verbal communication. The conversations that do take place do not involve the level of self-disclosure that is so often a part of general interchange among European American groups. Their conversation is a practice in self-restraint as they carefully avoid confrontational topics and subjects concerning the past which might be painful.

A new person who enters the environment of Kanriye's home or dance studio is never told not to talk too much, nor are they told that to discuss personal facts about their lives is inappropriate. However, everyone around her is observing a lesson quietly, finishing work on a *kimono* in silence, or watching the television without commenting on it. As I spent more and more time at the studio, the silence which was part of the environment became part of my life as well. I did not realize that I had come to accept it as a given until someone came into the environment with a different interpersonal style. A succession of these moments helped me to understand the changes which had taken place in my value system. I had come to appreciate the quiet communication and group belongingness that was part of my interaction while at the studio.

Japanese Americans studying with Kanriye Fujima have found reinforcement for a set of behaviors which are similar to those practiced at some level in their indigenous community. The training received through study with Kanriye Fujima reinforces social values that are an important aspect in understanding themselves as part of a community that shares a similar communicational style. The system of training traditional performers, whose manifest function both in Japan and in the United States is to maintain an art form, functions on a latent level in both countries to both develop and reinforce a set of personality traits that conforms to some experience of interpersonal styles of Japanese and Japanese Americans.

As De Vos and Romanucci-Ross point out, "For the individual, ethnicity is part of the gradual and continual definition of self that occurs as part of psychosexual development" (De Vos and Romanucci-Ross, 1975, p. 375). For all students, whether or not their forefathers came from Japan, the lessons with Kanriye Fujima are an opportunity for self-definition through encountering a form that is on some level different from their upbringing. The initial experience of taking lessons can be one of cultural shock as the students are, within the geographic boundaries of the United States, participating in the social interactions of a group that is on some level dissimilar to their previous experience. To be successful in the group the student must be able to overcome their initial reaction and duplicate the interactional patterns of the group. This experience of culture shock can according to Kim and Ruben have positive results. Basing their approach on the work of Adler, Kim and Ruben (1988) consider culture shock to be part of a positive learning experience from participating in a context outside of your personal background:

> In the intercultural communication-as-learning/growth approach, then, culture shock experiences are viewed as the core or essence, through not necessarily the totality, of the cross cultural learning experience. The culture-shock process is regarded as fundamental in that the individual must somehow confront the social, psychological, and philosophical discrepancies one finds between his or hew own internalized cultural disposition and that of the new environment. (Kim and Ruben, 1988, p. 304)

Kim and Ruben maintain that the adjustment for the individual is a two fold process of disorientation followed by a period of integration in which the individual has "restructured their internal conditions" (Kim and Ruben, 1988, p. 312). An individual, who has undergone one cultural shock experience, will if he/she encounters another such experience have an intuitive method of responding to it. Over time there is an increase in an individual's ability to be an effective intercultural communicator. In another article in the same volume, Collier and Thomas examine the relationship between intercultural communication and intercultural competence. They contend that people with a high degree of intercultural competence have had substantial opportunities to engage in intercultural communication and as a result see themselves as multi-cultural individuals who instead of belonging to a specific cultural group live on the boundaries while negotiating between groups.

Regardless of their ethnic backgrounds, students who began a course of study with Kanriye Fujima get an opportunity to expand their levels of experience through engaging in a sub-culture which to varying extent diverges from their own. This divergence varies not only along generational or ethnic lines, but the individual history of each student. Furthermore, their training provides the student with a set of psychophysical skills which may not directly relate to the inter-communicational style of their natal group. However, the nonverbal proficiency can become a useful observational tool in developing their ability to communicate interculturally. In a diverse society this degree of sensitivity could prove to be helpful in cross-cultural communication. It could be said that the students have developed a level of nonverbal sensitivity that may help them negotiate gracefully between groups.

The students acknowledge the importance the study of *buyo* has had in increasing their level of self-understanding. They do not necessarily draw parallels between their increased psychophysical abilities and the quality of their lives. I would argue that the increased somatic awareness on the part of the students allows them to more readily be aware of the nonverbal information that is part of any communicational interchange. The training in the studio, in which they must be able to follow increased amounts of subtle movement, is carried over into social interactions. This does not mean the student is always cognizant of the meaning of the nonverbal text only that she is more aware of it than she would have been without the training. For students who have studied *buyo* since childhood, it is an ability they assume is natural. Patsy Abe, a *Nisei* student who started serious study as an adult, identifies what she has learned as "a potential for living life effortlessly."

Nihon Buyo and its Communities in the Pacific Northwest

During Kanriye Fujima's life in the Pacific Northwest she has interacted with two different community groups; those who trace all or a portion of their ancestry to Japan and those who do not. Within each of these communities there have been people who have been students and others who have been audience. She has had the most direct influence on those people who have been students. However, she has had an indirect influence on audiences in all three communities. She has, as a transmitter of culture, a distinct relationship with each student group and the separate audiences in the three communities.

Each generational group in the Japanese American community has had a historically disparate relationship with Kanriye Fujima. For the *Issei*, especially the *Shin Issei* war brides who arrived in the United States following the occupation of Japan after World War II, she is someone who has shared a common experience. She speaks the same native language, shares memories of life in Japan, and understands from personal experience what it is like to be a stranger in a new country. They also have a common cultural basis for understanding the mutual responsibilities between teacher and student. For the *Nisei*, she is, through her teaching and performing, a living link between them and the world of their parents and grandparents. She personifies a Japan that many of them have never seen, but have heard about through stories told to them by their parents. For the *Sansei* and *Yonsei* (whether or not of interethnic heritage) she is the reverse of the Japan of technocrats depicted in the current mass media. She is for them a link to Japan's mythology and history.

The experience of the Japanese Americans as students and performers helps them to negotiate their personal ethnic identity along the exoteric (dominant culture) esoteric (ethnic group) continuum. The degree to which they are influenced by their study with Kanriye Fujima to an increased identification with their Japanese heritage varies depending upon generational affiliation, geographical location, and continued contact with their ancestral family in Japan. Those students who are first generation Japanese American, live an area such as Portland that is being increasingly influenced by Japanese economic life or have close ties with family in Japan, are the most likely to become deeply invested in the study of *nihon buyo* and the values associated with it. For instance, the *natori*

CHART 8-C

THE RELATIONSHIP BETWEEN THE NATORI,
THE COMMUNITIES, AND THE
PERFORMANCE CONTEXT

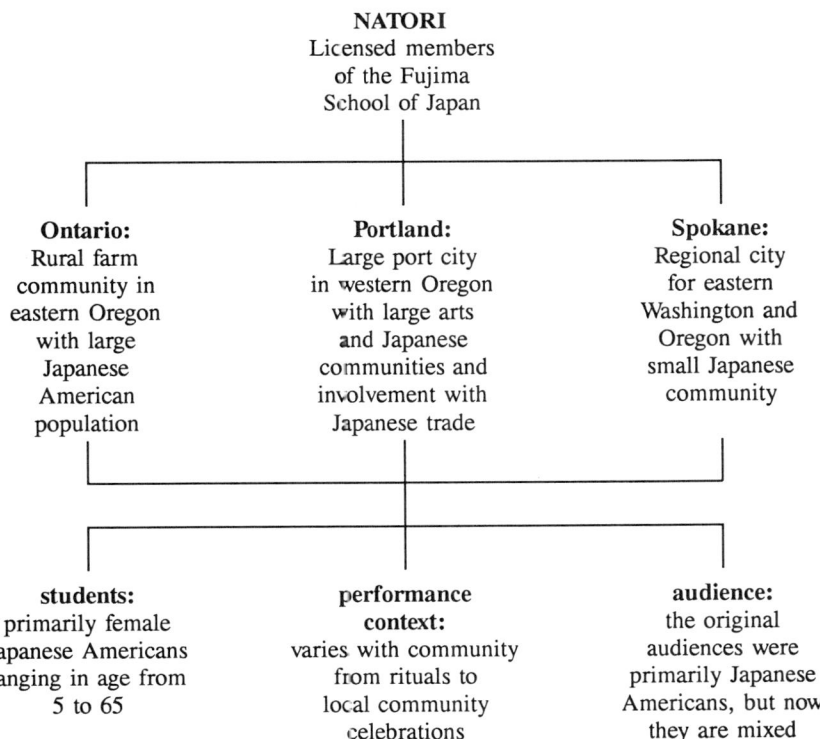

NATORI
Licensed members of the Fujima School of Japan

Ontario: Rural farm community in eastern Oregon with large Japanese American population

Portland: Large port city in western Oregon with large arts and Japanese communities and involvement with Japanese trade

Spokane: Regional city for eastern Washington and Oregon with small Japanese community

students: primarily female Japanese Americans ranging in age from 5 to 65

performance context: varies with community from rituals to local community celebrations

audience: the original audiences were primarily Japanese Americans, but now they are mixed

Lines represent potential for interchange.

and the other *Shin Issei*, like many of the original *Issei*, have developed a life style and social bonds around the study of an art form. The majority of the other students see each other only at lessons or performances. Recently, due to the increasing influence of Japan in the Pacific Northwest, some *Sansei* and interethnic students from Portland have continued to study past high school and have expressed an interest in becoming *natori*. Students who live in Ontario or Spokane, and are from interethnic families in which neither parent has any ties to Japan, are less likely to become as involved long term either in the schools or the related life style.

All students receive training and perform as part of one or another of the three communities' schools. Each school performs within its community at a variety of events. Each community focuses on different aspects of its Japanese American heritage but shares certain features that date from the beginning of Japanese settlement in the United States. The celebration of specific *matsuri* (festivals) have long been a part of Japanese American life in the United States. These festivals can be divided into two categories, public and private.[4] The most important private celebration takes place at New Year as people clean their homes, pay off old debts, prepare special foods, and spend three days visiting with friends in order to prepare themselves for the new year. Public celebrations take place in communities where there are sizable numbers of Japanese Americans. Consistently, one of the most important public *matsuri* has been *Obon* or the Buddhist festival in honor of the ancestors. The *Obon* dances held as part of the festival at Buddhist churches in Portland, Ontario, and Spokane are attended by many people who are not members of the regular Buddhist congregation. Other celebrations in honor of their heritage include Spokane's Japan Week in August and Portland's *Tanabata* in July.

Nihon buyo in the Pacific Northwest is not a direct transplant from Japan. An audience member at a *nihon buyo* concert in Portland will not necessarily witness a duplicate of a performance in Kyoto or Tokyo. A concert in Japan will generally feature older performers accompanied by on-stage musicians with elaborate costumes and stage settings. What the audience does see is a form continued within the *iemoto* system which includes performers moving to the same story lines and in costuming which is as close as the budget will allow to its Japanese counterpart.

The audiences have watched and heard the performances of primarily young children telling stories in movement of the young itinerant lion dancers of Echigo, the magnificence of the emperor compared to the glory of the chrysanthemum in *Kikuzukushi*, the world of the young geisha in *Maisugata*, the story of the bravery of young warrior in *Kuroda bushi*. They have as audience members participated in the complex stories of love and misfortune of heroes and heroines such as Goro and Onatsu. Traditional *sanbaso* pieces enacted by the more advanced students have recreated performances taken originally from the medieval *noh* theater as well as the Tokugawa-based *kabuki*. The beauty of the Japanese countryside and the gaiety of Japanese festivals have been depicted on stages at high schools, community centers, performing art centers, Japanese Gardens, and at Buddhist temples in Oregon and Washington.

The audiences in the three communities, although they may not have always shared the same context of performance, have had an opportunity to see the same dance/theater pieces performed. Audiences in Portland, beyond recitals, have seen presentations in combination with other arts groups within the community. Audiences in Spokane, beyond celebrations of Japanese American holidays, have seen presentations in combination with sister city programs. Audiences in Ontario have seen performances most often connected with *Obon* and other Buddhist celebrations.

The audience has changed over the thirty years from one of primarily Japanese with few non-Japanese to a mixed audience which includes people from a variety of ethnic backgrounds. This does vary, however, depending upon the event. The *Tanabata* Festival and the *Odori* night in Portland include people from diverse ethnic backgrounds. Their participation is limited more by financial means (can they afford the price of admission to the Japanese Gardens) than by ethnic status. But, the audience for the thirtieth anniversary recital held in 1987 at the Portland State University Theater was attended primarily by members of the Japanese American community. While the participants in the folk dances associated with the *Obon* Festival in Ontario are primarily Japanese Americans, the audience contains families of Japanese descent, a blend of Japanese/non-Japanese, European American and Mexican American parentage. The Sister City performance in Spokane had only a small number of Japanese Americans in comparison to the multi-ethnic blend of the entire audience. Thus, the current audience, with the exception of the thirtieth anniversary recital, has, for most performances, contained a wide variety people from the entire community. This has transformed what would ordinarily be considered ritual events (*Obon* and *Tanabata*) restricted to the ethnic community and thus could be considered a rite of cultural renewal to a celebration shared with the community at large of specific ethnic identity. The recital attended by primarily the ethnic community becomes the event at which the members acknowledge the skills and associated cultural knowledge of the students as reflected in their performances.

The Japanese American and non-Japanese audience was watching an enactment of a world with which neither was familiar. Even those Japanese American members of the audience who had been born in or visited Japan had probably never been to the Japan of *nihon buyo* with its ties to the flower and willow world of traditional theater. They came either from the rural countryside where they had been born or have visited the post-World War II Japan of tall buildings and crowded commuter trains. The audiences were watching performances directed by a person with her own image of Japan based in large part on the traditional world of Japanese theater. Kanriye Fujima has created a world on stage in the United States for non-Japanese and Japanese Americans of a Japan which is an interpretation of her theatrical experience.

Grounded in his examination of the history of persistent ethnic communities, anthropologist Edward Spicer (1971) has suggested groups continue because they share "a personal affiliation with certain symbols, or more accurately, with what certain symbols stand for" (Spicer 1971, p. 795). He contended that people continue to maintain their ethnic identity because members of the community continue to share a cumulative image, expressed symbolically, of a specific historical experience. The most successful of these symbols are those that have a built-in flexibility such as rituals and theater and whose associated elements of music and dance have an intense meaning for the people involved:

> The meanings amount to a self-definition and an image of themselves as they have performed in the course of their history. The selection of cultural elements for symbolic references goes on in terms of the character of this image; the frequent shifts in emphasis are part of the process of maintenance in response to alterations in the environment. (Spicer, 1971, p. 798)

The value of Spicer's model for a study of an individual life related to theater is that it incorporates several key ideas that are associated with both: the concept of identity as associated with the individual's conception of it rather than the historian's; the role of symbols in the maintenance of identity; and the use of ritual/theater in creating an environment that allows for the evolution and flexibility of the symbols.

Kanriye Fujima, a traveling dance teacher/performer, through her teaching and arrangement of performances, has served as a source of information for

American communities both Japanese American and otherwise to evolve their individual and community identity based on some understanding of their historical past as it has been incorporated into their historical present. She has also served as a broker between cultures by providing a means for Japanese Americans to participate in an aspect of traditional culture which has allowed them to explore as individuals to a greater or lesser degree the Japanese aspect of their personal heritage. She has produced *nihon buyo* performances within the varying contexts of the communities in the Pacific Northwest. She has provided contact between modern Japan and the United States in her close ties with the Fujima school. This continued relationship has made it possible for her to bring to the United States the most recent styles of *nihon buyo*. It has also made it possible for Japanese Americans to travel to Japan to become certified by the school. She has served as a teacher for the large communal dances of *Obon*. By accepting non-Japanese students she has participated in the enculturation of non-Japanese into a Japanese ethos. She has accomplished this through a traditional theatrical form that provides a system for teaching with built in potential for flexibility and strong visual images of Japanese mythology, culture, and history. The themes of the sung stories enacted by the students stress an individual's duty to family and community, the impermanence of life, and difficulties when one encounters separation from one's community.

Spicer argues that in order for an ethnic group to continue to maintain its identity, the group must hold in common a strong shared image that is part of the ritual and theater associated with the group. From the early twentieth century with the arrival of female immigrants from Japan, there have been women trained in some form of dance or theater who have helped in teaching the community the folk dances associated with *Obon*. Since World War II, there have been women trained in *nihon buyo* who have taught members of the community, most often young girls and women, the *nihon buyo* pieces that would be performed within the same event.

Kanriye Fujima has been the vehicle for the shared image of Japanese culture among all community groups through the image of the young Japanese girl or woman in the costume and make-up of the Tokugawa era theater. When Kanriye Fujima first arrived in the United States thirty-two years ago, the newspaper accounts of recitals included a picture of a young woman (Kanriye Fujima) in traditional costume. Today announcements of performances have continued to feature a photograph of an elaborately kimono clad Japanese girl or woman in a three dimensional pose. In 1988, the Ontario newspaper, *The Daily Argus*, used a large photograph of women dancers at *Obon* as the cover for its special

Thursday section on the upcoming festival. There has been almost no important event in any of the three Japanese American communities in which a female figure clad in traditional garb was not part of the event. In some cases, such as the Japan Week celebration in Spokane in August of 1989, it was the event around which the rest of the week was planned.

Within the interplay of the dance pieces and the context in which it has been presented, this figure has become what Sherry Ortner refers to as a summarizing symbol. These symbols "are seen as summing up, expressing, representing for the participants in an emotionally powerful and relatively undifferentiated way, what the system means to them" (Ortner, 1979, p. 94). The kimono clad Japanese female performer seems to represent for Japanese American communities in the Pacific Northwest both the country from which they came and the life their families have created in America. This life only developed into established communities with the arrival of the women who as wives and mothers helped in the formation of families, and who as teachers of traditional arts helped to maintain a variation of a Japanese sensibility in the United States.

Author Mike Thiele in his book titled *Footprints Across Oregon* dedicates an entire chapter to Kanriye Fujima entitling it "The Traditionalist." This phrase understates the complex role which Kanriye Fujima plays within the communities in which she teaches. Her sphere of influence includes Americans of both Japanese and non-Japanese descent in three separate communities. This larger group can further be divided into those who are or have been students and those who are members of the audience. Kanriye Fujima and the dance/theater she teaches symbolize Japan to members of these communities whether or not they are of Japanese descent. The *nihon buyo* performances, either as part of a concert or a local celebration in one of the three communities, have been until recently the primary visual image of Japan for many non-Japanese as well as Japanese Americans.

This complex symbol associated as it is with the social history of Japanese in both Japan and the United States has a multiplicity of meanings for students and audience. It includes a system of training and the attendant nonverbal skills associated with it. Through the actual performance, key scenarios of the duty of individuals to family and group are reinforced by Japanese mythology and history. This is augmented by specific images from nature. All students of *nihon buyo* are transformed through the process of training and performance into a symbol of Japanese culture. This symbol especially when portrayed by another Japanese American transports the Japanese Americans watching to their roots within the communities in which they were raised. To the non-Japanese audience the symbol becomes their understanding of what it means to be culturally Japanese.

Kanriye Fujima: Cultural Transmitter

Kanriye Fujima's public persona is a blend of Japan and America but with an emphasis placed on her Japanese heritage. The majority of her students, especially those in Portland and Spokane, except for school social events, see her dressed only in the *kimono* in which she teaches. Although she may give the young students a lollipop at the end of a lesson, she still expects aspects of their behavior while at lessons to conform to her interpretation and application of Japanese etiquette. Her conversations with them are a combination of Japanese and English with a heavy emphasis on Japanese. Pictures of her which have appeared in brochures, programs, and newspapers in all three communities show her attired in some form of *nihon buyo* costume or other Japanese dress.

Her life reveals a woman who is committed to living a life which is rooted in a specific artistic heritage and yet who is capable of adapting her life and the form to meet the changing needs of the community. She prefers in her private life to surround herself with as many aspects of Japan as is possible even while living in the United States. She has also surrounded herself with women who share her dedication to the art form she teaches.

Kanriye Fujima's approach to teaching and performing in the United States fits Kitano's comparison of the adaptation process of Japanese Americans in general:

> The Japanese themselves like to compare it to a small stream; like a stream they have followed the contours of the land, followed the lines of least resistance, avoided direct confrontation, and developed at their own pace, always shaped by the external realities of the larger society. (Kitano, 1976, p. 3)

Like a flowing stream Kanriye Fujima, in her teaching and programs, has maintained a consistency of teaching method while changing the dance pieces taught in response to the shifts in the audience for which they were intended. The students have always been taught with tolerance and gentle persuasion but were and are expected to follow the strict dress and deportment associated with Japanese traditional art forms. She has adapted the *iemoto* system acting as a strong head of the respective schools, always making all decisions related to the running of them. This includes where and when she will teach, where and when the groups will perform, what pieces will be performed and what costumes will be worn. Yet, she has not exercised the same control over the natori's lives as would a teacher of the form in Japan. Like a stream she maintained the course in those areas of her teaching and performing which fit well within the culture in which she was living. However, when necessary she changed course in those areas which accommodated her students and the audiences of her adopted country.

The care and devotion which Sensei gives to teaching each student some aspects of Japanese culture during lessons and performances is returned in the appreciation the students feel towards her. This is especially true as they get older. Diana Snell, a college student, has felt that "Sensei always encourages everyone at whatever skill level they have." Karla, a former student while in high school student, said "I started late and felt clumsy, but Sensei always made me feel alright about what I was doing." Diane Hinatsu, a graduate of Oregon State University and performer with several modern dance companies in the Portland area, has credited Sensei with her understanding of the relationship between dance and life. Amy, a new six year old student, just feels good being at lessons with Sensei. All of them can not imagine taking lessons with any other teacher.

Except for Native American populations, the United States has evolved as a nation of immigrants. Until the 1960s, there was an attempt on the part of the Western European majority to encourage new immigrants from Eastern Europe and elsewhere to adopt their way of life. The ethnic theater of the United States reflects this trend. The themes of the plays of many ethnic theaters in the late nineteenth and early twentieth century focused on methods of adapting to life in the United States. As these groups became assimilated, the majority of the theaters disappeared. The exceptions to this trend were the Jewish and Black theaters which for their respective communities contained strong religious and cultural symbols. (Seller, 1983)

The civil rights movement of the 1960s helped to redefine political policy in regard to attempts to turn the United States into a melting pot. There was an increased emphasis on ethnic awareness. This was the beginning of the study of Black American, Mexican American, Native American, and Asian American theater. These theaters have, for the most part, combined various elements from the long history of western theater to create productions that thematically speak to the life issues experienced by each population group. In the 1980s, it has become popular both in the United States and Japan to blend Japanese and Western theater to create *kabuki* or *noh* versions of western classics. *Nihon buyo*, as it has been taught and produced by Kanriye Fujima in the Pacific Northwest, runs counter to both of these trends. It is a continuation in the United States of a theater form that traces its origins to seventh century Japan.

Kanriye Fujima is just one of many *nihon buyo* teachers on the west coast of the United States. She is part of the Asian theater in general and other aspects of Asian culture that are impacting the United States as there is a shift in the balance of world power. She is a teacher in the modern era of mass transportation and communication. Thirty-two years ago when she came to the United States she arrived by a slow boat across the Pacific; she now flies from Oregon to Tokyo in less than a day. Video tapes were not part of the mass culture when she left Japan. She now watches taped television programs from Japan. She uses the video tape as an aid in teaching and to evaluate student performances.

The study of Kanriye Fujima's life in dance/theater in the United States indicates that, at least in one instance, an artist trained in a traditional form has immigrated to a new country, taught the form in the adopted country, and yet maintained strong ties with her country of origin. In Japan she is one of the respected students of Kansho Fujima and as such fulfills the set of role expectations associated with that position. When she is in the United States, she is head of schools that with some variation operate within the same general structure. Her ability to be successful in both worlds is an indication of her ability to negotiate between two separate cultures. Her teaching in this country has encouraged Japanese Americans to maintain ties with the artistic traditions of the country of their ancestors. Without both elements--her teaching in the United States and consistent trips to Japan--those students who so desired would not have been able to go to Japan to become *natori*. Although the only members of the school who have taken advantage of Kanriye Fujima's ties to the Fujima school in Japan have been *Shin Issei* current *Sansei* or *Yonsei* students may decide to become *natori*.

Kanriye Fujima is part of a vast intercultural exchange between ethnic groups in the United States and the countries from which they came, an exchange that is increased because of the ease of modern communication. Her teaching is an example of the interplay between aesthetic and social drama both on a personal and national level. A Japanese dramatic form was reconstructed in the Pacific Northwest because a woman trained in the traditional system wanted to have the expressive independence she had experienced in Japan due to war with the United States. Her life in the Pacific Northwest has allowed her to engage in many aspects of the form that would not have been possible in Japan. Nevertheless, she has continued the principal elements of the form and system in which she was trained.

Notes

1. The interrelationship between social and aesthetic drama has been discussed by Victor Turner and Richard Schechner in a number of different articles. These include: Turner, *The Anthropology of Performance*, (New York: PAJ, 1986); Schechner, *Performance Theory*, (New York: Routledge, 1988); and, Schechner and Appel, eds., *By Means of Performance* (New York: Cambridge University Press, 1990).

2. Kanriye Fujima is not the only Japanese artist since World War II to seek greater expressive freedom in the United States. An article discussing this subject is: "In Japan, Huddled Masses Yearning to be Free," *Los Angeles Times* Monday, June 29, 1992:A12-A13.

3. They would, however, ask Kanriye Fujima's permission to teach. They also do not make decisions about which pieces will be performed; they only insure that the program takes place.

4. A good description of material culture of Japanese American communities in the United States is in Haseltine (1989).

APPENDIX A

THE DANCES AND PROGRAM NOTES OF

FUJINAMI-KAI

The Portland school, Fujinami-kai, has kept since 1957 two forms of records: a set of programs from recitals and formal performances; and a card file of dances performed in informal spaces for which there is no program. The following are the dances and program notes of Fujinami-kai as the members themselves have recorded them. I have not tried to alter or elaborate upon them. However in cases of slightly different descriptions, I have rewritten the information to reflect both.

A Hiroshima

This deeply sensitive number is a prayer dedicated to the rebuilt city of Hiroshima after the devastation of the atomic bomb during World War II. The people of the city renewed with hope for the future pray for eternal peace among all nations.

A Tabarugaka
(A Historical Dance of the end of the Feudal Era set in Kyushu)

The background story of this number is the war between the feudal power and advocates for Japan's awakening. The warriors of the central government have overwhelmed the young soldiers of Saigo Takamori, the leader fighting to preserve old samurai values. This dance tells of their last stand as they write their wills knowing that they will be slain.

Agari sai no hana
This is a modern piece in which the singer is explaining the parallels between the beauty of a flower and the beauty of his love.

Aikawa ondo
This folk song tells the story of a young samurai warrior who longs to display his bravery and skill in war. The song comes from Niigata in Northern Japan. It tells the story of a Japanese hero Yoshitsune who while still in his early teens showed great bravery and skill in war.

Aizome gasa
Yakuza is a good for nothing bandit of the past. He is very brave in fights and quite clever at gambling. Because he leads such a life, he must always be away from his loved ones. As he dances he wishes that he could mend his ways and be with his love.

Aki no irokusa
(The Colored Grasses of Autumn)

This dance taken from the kabuki theater is a classical number praising the beauty of autumn flowers. The dancers are young maid servants in the employ of a princess.

Amagai goe
(Beautiful Amagai)

This dance describes the beauty of Amagai an area south of Tokyo.

Amagasa karakasa
(Umbrella)

On a rainy day, children carrying umbrellas go down to the station to meet their father coming home from the city. Holding high their brightly colored umbrellas, they try to signal their father as he searches for them in the crowd.

Amano yari rihei

This dance tells the story of a sword maker who secretly forged weapons for a famous battle. Suspected of disloyalty for his activities, even his family was harassed by the authorities, but he remained loyal to his friends.

Ame furi otsukisan
(Rain Moon a Children's Song)

When it rains the moon is hidden behind the clouds while a young woman is getting ready to be married. She rides to her wedding in a carriage. The horses must hurry or dawn will break and the moon-bride will disappear.

Ame no bojo
(Longings)

The rain reminds a woman of her former lover. In her loneliness she longs for his companionship. The mixed feelings associated with their separation are forgotten.

Ame no goro
(Goro in the Rain)

Goro is one of two brothers who avenges the death of their father who had been killed 18 years before in a private quarrel. Their enemy has come to be a powerful governor. Their task is not an easy one. Both brothers are killed after they accomplish their purpose. Of the two brothers, Goro is the rash one--always rushing into fights.

Aobajo koi uta
(Green Leaf Castle Love Song)

This is the theme of Tanabata and is a popular ballad. A singer strolling along gazing at the summer stars, thinking of a lover. The Tanabata decorations are everywhere, but the lover will no longer return.

Aoyagi
(Green Willow)

The mood of this dance is romantic. As a dancer gazes out into a garden, she sees the silhouette of her lover in the shadows of a weeping willow. However, on closer inspection she realizes that what she sees is only the reflection of the moon. On another occasion, she hears her lover calling softly, but closer attention reveals that a parrot is mimicking her lover's voice. The sad truth is she is alone and very lonely.

Asadoya yunta
A folk song from Okinawa, a small island at the southern end of Japan.

Awayuki gonpachi
This tells of a handsome fugitive who is being pursued by the authorities. Hidden under an umbrella he walks through the snow to secretly meet his geisha girl friend.

Ayame sendo
This dance tells the story of several geisha pretending to be boatmen. As they row they sing of the lovely iris blooming in Itako.

Ayame yukata
(Summer Silhouette)

This is a dance of the summer season. Two geisha clad in their summer kimono which are gaily patterned with iris flowers are seen as they express the seasonal changes of summer in Japan.

Ayatsuri sanbaso
The performer is imitating the movements of a marionette.

Bankokuhaku ondo
This dance commemorates the fabulous Expo 70 that was held in Osaka.

Beni higasa
(Crimson Parasol)

This is a story of a daughter of a weaver, a very talented dancer. She is coming home from a visit to a shrine, when she joins a group of professional dancers. The girl dances so gracefully and so skillfully that she far outshines the professional performers that are entertaining at the shrine.

Bura bura bushi
(Festive Dance of Nagasaki)

This dance tells the story of a girl out for a stroll during festival time. She meets many people in a gay, holiday mood. Among them is a drunkard who goes staggering along the road. As the girl continues her walk, it begins to rain so she protects her head with her apron. The strap of her wooden clogs breaks and she limps hurriedly home.

Byakko no shiro
(A Feudal Castle of Fukushima)

A Buddhist priest comes to visit the graves of the young warriors who died during a historic battle loyally defending their lord's castle.

Byakkotai
(Dance of the Samurai)

The youths of the White Tiger Brigade died to the last man, in the hopeless defense of the Tokugawa Shogun. One last survivor fights his way out of battle, climbs a hill, and sees his castle consumed in flames in the valley below. He recalls his friends in battle, and finally joins them in death.

Chakkiri bushi
(Women of the Tea Leaves)

On the hillsides of Shizuoka, women are picking tea leaves. As they are busily at work, they hear frogs in the nearby swamps begin to croak. This is said to be a sign for rain the next day. The women hurry with their picking hoping that the omen is not true because there is more work to do tomorrow.

Chanchiki okesa
(Memories of Home)

Far from home, this traveler stops to enjoy a cup of rice wine, sake. As he drinks, nostalgic memories of home, family and a former sweetheart make him sad and lonely.

Chiyo gami no hana
(Paper Flower)

These dancers are folding colored papers into many shapes. There are delicate peach blossoms for the peach festival, there are pears for the August moon celebration, and for New Year's shiny gold and silver flowers are made. These varied shapes are interpreted by the use of two fans.

Cho cho
(Butterflies)

Children watching the butterflies in delight, telling the butterflies to go this way and then that way.

Daishobu
(A Magnificent Victory)

This is a creed for a life, for a man to be victorious, to love and to be free from regrets. The creed for a woman is to be respected, to be loyal and to be humble. For both it is to value life but to give up one's life willingly for friendship and loyalty. To live from day to day upholding this creed is the goal of the Japanese way of life.

Don don bushi

This was a popular song of medieval Japan. It is divided into 3 parts: a historical ballad, a love story, and a rice wine drinking song.

Don pan bushi

This is a folk dance from the Akita prefecture. Dancers step to the sounds of rice being threshed after a rice harvest. This number is adapted to modern music and the girls are wearing mini kimono.

Echigo jishi
(Lion Dancers of Edo)

These performers are performing the lion dance in the streets from the county of Echigo or Edo (former Tokyo). The lion denotes good luck, endurance and strength. This dance is performed on festive occasions. The tempo of the fast rhythm is very difficult to maintain, and the most difficult section is the last part, where the dancers manipulate the long, white cloth to the fast tempo of the music.

Echigo jishi no uta
(Song of the Lion's dance)

An unscrupulous man uses orphan children to beg for money. These dancers are performing the song of the Lion's dance in the street hoping that the people will throw coins. If they go back empty-handed, the orphans must again be subjected to beatings from their cruel master.

Ehi gasa
(The Parasol Dance)
This is a children's dance displaying their talents with a parasol.

Fuji
This is a traditional dance that is performed by odori students studying for their teaching certificates. All movements of classical dancing are included in this number.

Fuji murasaka
(Lavender Wisteria)
In Japanese classical dance, one of the most colorful, popular numbers is Fuji musume (The Maiden of Wisteria.) Fuji murasaka, taken from the Fuji musume is a new arrangement of Yamato Gaku, which is a modern interpretation of Japanese classical music. The dance depicts beautiful clusters of wisteria blossoms swaying under a trellis of wisteria vines, and butterflies playing among the rich, lavender wisteria. This is one of the most popular maiden dances included in the Yamato Gaku.

Fuji musume
(Wisteria Maiden)
A beautiful girl carrying a wisteria spray under a pine entwined in wisteria-- this is perhaps the most popular image in buyo dance. The wisteria spirit loves the pine, but he is indifferent. The dance shows a young woman's love in its many forms--playful and serious, shy and flirtatious, hopeful and despairing, forgiving and angry. The Wisteria Maiden is a true classic, a transformation piece requiring the mastery of many different techniques and moods.

Fuji no hana
(Wisteria Blossoms)
Our dance school which is called the Fujima School has for its symbol or crest, the graceful wisteria blossom. This dance expresses the essence and beauty of this flower.

Fuji-san
This dance is in praise of the beauty of the perfect cone shape of Mt. Fuji. This splendid mountain presents various aspects of beauty--snow covered starkness in the winter and classic splendor against the blue sky.

Fukagawa
(Ballad)

This number is in three parts. The first shows two oarsmen on a sightseeing boat on the Fukagawa, a river in Tokyo. In the second part, two hand held carriers are on their way to Yoshiwara. And in the final part, two monks are having a gay time in a wine shop.

Funakata-san
(Ferry Boatmen)

This is a spirited dance of the hard working boatmen who ferry people across the river.

Genroku hanami odori
(Cherry Blossom Dance)

The Genroku period corresponds to the year 1688-1703 of the Christian era. The country was a peace and prosperous and most kabuki dances were developed at this time. The cherry blossom time is a festive occasion and these girls stepping out of the ancient Genroku era are dancing under the lovely cherry blossoms.

Gion kouta
(Ballad of Gion)

Gion is the district in Kyoto where the Maiko community lives. These dancers are apprentice geisha called Maiko. Dancing under the cherry blossoms, they tell about their work: dancing, singing, playing an instrument, practicing calligraphy, arranging flowers, executing the tea ceremony. All of these are part of their profession as paid entertainers.

Gojoobashi

This is one of the adventures of Ushiwaka Maru, a son of a famous feudal lord. Benkei, a giant warrior-priest is collecting 1000 swords as his contribution to a temple. He has taken 999 swords by force and the 1000th belongs to Ushiwaka Maru. Benkei challenges the young boy of twelve on the Gojoobashi (gojoo bridge) thinking him an easy conquest. A struggle follows and the boy overcomes the priest. The priest surrenders meekly and promises to become a faithful follower of Ushiwaka Maru. Ushiwaka Maru, whose real name was Minamoto Yoshitsune was a famous warrior who lived in the twelfth century. His adventures supplied material for many Japanese plays, poetry and novels. He was also one of the most colorful men in Japanese history.

Goman goku
During the historic feudal days this particular section of Japan called Goman was not a prosperous place but it was very beautiful. The dance extols the many natural beauty spots of the local.

Goro tokimune
(Goro, the Samurai)

This is an old legendary tale of the great samurai or warrior, Goro, who had the reputation of being very temperamental and hot headed. His father had been murdered but Goro hides his feelings and waits for the opportune time to take revenge.

Goshugi kotobuki sanba
Traditionally, all kabuki dramas and dance programs are opened with this stylized type of ceremonial number. This dance clears the air of all evil so that good luck and good cheer will prevail for the evening. In the kabuki, the dance is performed by a male actor.

Gosho guruma
(Festivity Dance)

This is a semi-classical dance in the romantic vein. These lovers are in the service of a lord's household. Strict regulations forbid them from expressing their personal feelings or emotions. And so, these lovers, communicate with one another by means of writing poetry and by dancing.

Gyo sen
(Sailor's Dance--Niigata)

This is a very spirited dance about fishermen who are rowing their boat sailing out into the sea for a day's catch of fish. The performers use a wooden paddle to depict the movements of the dance.

Hakata yobune
This story takes place at a harbor on the island of Kyushu. A lovely geisha stands by the water waiting the arrival of the boat on which her lover is coming.

She stands quietly wondering when the boat will arrive and whether the boat is on a sea which is calm or stormy.

Hana
(Flowers)

The art of flower arranging is part of the training of cultured Japanese women. In this number, the dancers are making flower arrangements. The blossoms awaken lovely dreams of long ago. And as each stalk is carefully placed, beautiful thoughts sweep through the mind, for indeed the floral art helps to make the women's spirit more feminine and lovely.

Hanakage
(In the Shade of the Flowering Cherry)

A dance of two young girls beneath the flowers.

Hanami dojoji
(Flowers of Dojoji)

A dance of young girls looking at the flowers of Dojoji temple.

Hana no byakko tai

The background of this number tells of a group of nineteen young warriors about fifteen years of age from the locale of Fukushima. They have battled the enemy courageously but are defeated. Their lord's castle has been burned and many of their comrades have died. In the traditional way of honor among the warriors, they commit suicide or "hara-kiri."

Hana no orizuru gasa

A gambler, a man of fortune, must wander where chance beckons him. Consequently, he has no permanent relationships--he has no home, nor can he dare to fall in love with a woman.

Hana to ryuu

This too is a gambler's story. The spirit of sacrificing himself-giving his life for his friends or his master is told in this dance. On his back is tattooed the character, Ryuu, which symbolizes strength and courage.

Hana yome kitsune

This children's song tells of a disguised fox. In Japanese folklore, the fox disguises himself in many forms and hoodwinks many people. In this story, the fox is disguised as a bride. He is powdered and wigged and dressed beautifully. He is enjoying himself in this bridal role until he discovers that his tail is showing under the hem of his kimono. The people laugh at him and he runs back to the hills greatly embarrassed.

Hana yome ningyo

A bridal doll dressed beautifully in her traditional wedding kimono is sad because she must leave her family. However, she dares not cry for her tears would ruin her paper gown.

Hanafubuki dojoji
(Flowers of Dojoji)

These lovely maidens are out viewing the beautiful flowers in the garden of the Dojoji temple.

Hane no kamuro
(New Year's Feather Game)

The girls are playing battledore and shuttlecock, a game somewhat like our badminton. This game is played on New Year's, a very important holiday in Japan. The very elaborate and colorful costumes worn by the girls and the gay spirits of all make this a festive occasion.

Harimaya bashi
(Harimaya Bridge Kochi, Shikoku)

This tells the story of a priest who is attracted to a girl. Harimaya is the name of the bridge he crosses everyday to visit her. But, he neglects his religious duties and he is stripped of his religious robes and sent from the temple with just one umbrella. However, he is not sad because he knows that religious life is not for him. The worldly life beckons him too strongly.

Harukaze soran
(Fishermen's Dance)

This dance is from Hakkaido.

Haru no shirabe
(Spring Melody)

This is a congratulatory dance and is performed on happy occasions. The dancers in their colorful kimono portray the beautiful sights of springtime. It is the season when birds are singing and flowers are blooming.

Harusame
(Spring Rain)

A lovely geisha gazes upon a spring scene after the rain. Plum blossoms glisten with the raindrops and the humming birds quietly sing. It is an exquisite moment of loneliness and wonder.

Harusame jishi
(A Lion Dancer in the Spring rain)

In Japan on festive days, lion dancers perform for the crowds. The lion symbolizes endurance, strength, and good luck. This particular dance number portrays the life of such a lion dancer as he goes about in the spring rain.

Hashi zukushi
(Famous Bridges of Tokyo)

This song tells of the many famous bridges of Tokyo.

Hauta and Nidai

This is two dances. The first dance is: Waga Mono: A winter song in which the dancer does not feel the weight of the snow on her umbrella but the weight of the love in her heart.

The second dance is: Kasane Oogi: A dancer with many fans gazes at the plum and chrysanthemum blossoms. She feels very fortunate to be in such lovely surroundings. She expresses her happiness with the fans, spreading them out to show the breadth of good luck.

Hie tsuki bushi

This is a folk dance from the island of Kyushu. In the feudal days of Japan when the clans of Genji and Heike were in a civil war, the remnants of the defeated Heike samurai took refuge in Kyushu. Having no rice to eat they had to substitute a grain known as Hie. This is the dance in which the hard grain cover is pounded off.

Hie tsuki monogatari
(Ballad of a Defeated Samurai)
In the feudal days of Japan, a defeated samurai in retreat, grinding and pounding rice for his livelihood, reminisces his glorious past.

Hiroshima kiyari ondo
The group dance to a song originally sung happily by a group of lumbermen as they hauled lumber.

Hiroshima ondo
This lively number tells the story of the city of Hiroshima that was destroyed by the atom bomb during World War II. The city has since been rebuilt into a very modern city. The young people are dancing in the spirit of hope and prosperity.

Hisame
(Freezing Rain)
A woman is standing in the freezing rain thinking of her last love.

Hoo no mai
(Dance of the Phoenix)
Congratulatory number often used in the opening of a program.

Horete kayou
(Unrequited Love)
A young man travels to court to see the girl he loves, but unhappily she does not return his love.

Hotaru
(Firefly)
In Japan, the summer evening brings out many fireflies. It is an old traditional pastime for children to go firefly-catching.

Ina bushi
This folk dance tells of a ride down the swift Tenryu River on a raft. The raftsmen are wishing that they had an umbrella to protect them from the heavy spray.

Isami bune
Isami bune is a sturdy fishing boat that weathers the storms and high seas and gale-like winds. It departs with the crew anticipating a good catch and returns with men anticipating a joyous reunion with their loved ones.

Ise ondo
This is one of the many folk dances that make up the fabric of Japanese culture. This ondo is a dance of happiness telling of the wonders of Ise, the oldest shrine of Japan.

Issunboshi
(Tom Thumb)
In the Japanese version of Tom Thumb, Issunboshi bids farewell to his parents to go out into the world to seek his fortune. He sails down the river in a wooden bowl using chopsticks as oars. On an island he attempts to save a beautiful princess from a terrible demon, but instead he is eaten by the demon. Issunboshi inside the demon's stomach, stabs him with his sword which in truth is a needle. The demon coughs up Issunboshi and retreats leaving behind a magic wand. The princess makes a wish with the wand praying that Issunboshi would become tall and handsome. The wish is fulfilled, the couple marry and they live happily ever after.

Itako dejima
This is a folk dance of Itako, a locale noted for its beauty. The lovely iris flowers are in bloom and girls are dancing amid the flowers.

Itako koigasa
This dance tells the story of a young girl who rows her boat over the water where lovely iris flowers grow. Perhaps her lover, who has left the village, will return soon, perhaps not, but she will wait here.

Itako kuzushi
This story tells about a boatwoman of Itako. She is taking a bride to her new home, and is envious of the bride's happiness.

Itsuki no komori uta
A poor village girl is hired as a baby sitter in the city of Itsuki. With the baby strapped on her back, she goes outdoors to play. A group of wealthy

neighbor children come out and the little girl asks to join in their games, they tease and taunt her and the little girl begins to cry. Her clothes are shabby, she is treated badly and she is terribly lonely and homesick.

Itsuki yuyake
(Dusk at Itsuki-Kumamoto)

In farming localities in Japan, many young girls are hired out as baby sitters to help with the family's finances. This story tells of a young baby sitter who works for another family far from home. As dusk approaches she sees the setting sun, the young girl becomes very homesick and longs for her mother.

Itsuki no komori ningyo
(The Baby Sitter Doll)

This doll is in the image of a baby sitter, a poor village girl who is hired out by a wealthy family with the baby strapped on her back. She goes out to play but is teased and taunted by the other children. Her clothes are shabby, she is treated badly and she is terribly lonely and homesick.

Janome no kage de
(Under an Umbrella)

Hidden under the shade of a rain umbrella, a lovely girl weeps sadly of a broken heart. She has been rejected by the boy she loves. A tiny sparrow peers under the edge of the umbrella and advises her to forget him. There are many more just as handsome and charming.

Jinsei gekijo

This is a popular song praising the virtues of an honorable man.

Judo ichi dai
(The True Spirit of Judo)

This is a the dance translating the true spirit of Judo.

Jugo ya otsuki sama

These little girls are watching the beautiful full moon and recalling memories that are very sad.

Junrei otsuru
(A Tiny Pilgrim)

This is a tragic story of a little orphan girl Otsuru. She learns that her parents are living and sets out on a search to find them. During her wanderings throughout the countryside, she is recognized by her mother. Unfortunately, the parents are on an important mission of great secrecy and cannot disclose their true identity to their child. And so Otsuru continues on her endless search.

Jyu san ya
(The Night of the 13th)

Two nights before the moon is full, it is believed to be a very sad time. These dancers are viewing the moon and talking about their former loves.

Kabuki odori

A seven year old daughter of a kabuki star is very mature and precocious for her young years. The adults enjoy teasing her as she searches for a suitable boyfriend. This is a traditional number in the Fujima School, which all young dancers must master before they advance to the next level.

Kabuto
(A Warrior's Helmet)

The history of a warrior's helmet is related in this number. The battles both victorious and lost are recalled from the helmet's standpoint.

Kagura men
(A Comic Dance of Three Masks)

This is a comic number that employs the skillful handling of three masks. The story is the problem of the eternal triangle in the course of love. There are two boys and a girl. The girl prefers one boy and the rejected one becomes jealous.

Kaguyahime
(The Shinning Princess)

This is a well known Japanese fairy tale. An old man makes his living cutting bamboo trees. One day when he chops down a golden colored bamboo, he finds a baby girl. While she grows to be a lovely princess, the fortune of the old man improves and he becomes a rich man. When the princess is of marriageable age, she must return to the moon from which she came leaving the old man sad and lonely.

Kai no umekawa

Chubei, an employee in a government money exchange office, embezzles money to buy Umekawa, a geisha, before she is sold to someone else. This crime is punishable by death so the two run away to commit suicide.

Kami ningyo
(A Paper Doll)

A story of a paper doll who went out in the rain and got wet. She caught a cold but hates to take medicine.

Kami uri
(A Paper Vender)

The paper vender carries various kinds of paper used by Japanese families, which she sells on the street. She expresses by her dance, the old traditional festivals and holidays in each of the twelve months of the year.

Kanashii sake
(Sad Sake)

She tries to forget her love affair by drinking sake. But the more she drinks the more lonesome she becomes. She cannot forget her sad, sad, romance.

Kappore

This is a comic dance of a boatmen who is steering a boat loaded with oranges.

Kasabutai
(Dance in Two Parts)

The first part of this dance tells of the bamboo sprouts, a delicacy of the Japanese table. The dancers show how the sprouts grow day by day in the light of the sun and the light of the moon.

The second part is a parasol dance. There are different varieties of parasols, for rain, for mist, and for the sun. The dancers make a picturesque scene as they parade over the bridge.

Kawaii sakanaya san
(A Little Fish Vender)

This is a children's song depicting a fish vender coming around the town to sell fresh fish.

How do you do?
Would you like some fish today?
No? Then I'm on my way to another house.
I have all kinds and I'll cut them in size.
Well, I've sold all my fish for today.
Thank-you all and I'll see you tomorrow.

Kii no kuni
The province of Kii is famous for its many shrines. The shrine of the fox is the theme of this number.

Kiku no sakae
This is a ceremonial or congratulatory number that is the beginning of a Nihon Buyo presentation. It combines the imagery of the chrysanthemums, the emblem of the imperial family with references to patriotism.

Kikuzukushi
(Chrysanthemum Dance)

This is a dance of Chrysanthemum fairies, presenting different varieties of chrysanthemums. The chrysanthemum is the national flower of Japan. It includes eight little girls.

Kinno harusama gasa
This story is based on a historical event. The geisha, Ikumatsu, works as a spy for a political faction. She carries letters from her lover to his political friends.

Kira no nikichi
(A Man's Revenge)

Kira is a man who has a very strong sense of right and wrong. When his wife's brother commits an evil act, Kira feels that he must take the law on himself and punish his brother-in-law. Before he does, however, Kira divorces his wife and sends her home to her family in order that he will not disgrace her. Kira is eventually killed by his former brother-in-law.

Kiso bushi

Kiso bushi is a folk song from Nagano just north of Tokyo. It is a lively song of the river men who float rafts of logs down from the forest to the mills. The women at home worry about their menfolks on the river because it is very cold.

Kiso bushi sando gasa

This is a folk song of the logging country in Nagano. A logger turns into a gambler and travels over the countryside pursuing lady luck. He becomes homesick for his former home. He longs to see his girl friend. He misses the village children, but such is the loneliness of a gambler's life.

Kitsune bi
(Magic Fire)

A young lady learns that her family plans to kill her fiance for political reasons. She wishes to warn him, but the lake she must cross to reach him is dangerous with floating ice. While praying for help before a shrine, a fox tail on a helmet hanging nearby shines with a strange light exerting magical powers. The lake becomes frozen solid and the girl is able to cross over to warn her fiance in time.

Kiyoi jishi

An annual festival of dancers who are led by the lion dancers. In Japan this festival is sponsored annually by the firemen of the village.

Kocho no mai
(Dance of the Butterflies)

Butterflies fluttering among the red and white peonies welcome the arrival of spring. The furitsuzumi is used to produce the fast rhythm toward the end of the dance.

Koi no umegawa
(Passion of Umegawa)

This dance represents winter.

Kojo
(Feudal Castle)

Kojo tells the story of a samurai--a warrior of old feudal Japan. In his old age, the samurai visits the feudal castle where in his prime he served loyally under a renowned lord. As the samurai gazes at the castle which is crumbling into ruins from neglect, he recalls the prosperity of this fortress once long ago which has bittersweet memories.

Kojo shiragiku
(Girl of Devotion)

A tragic search for a lost father by his daughter is the story told in this dance. Along lonesome roads, over treacherous mountains, the girl travels with the hope of finding her father to fulfill her devotion to him.

Kokaji
(The Honorable Way of the Sword)

These dance acknowledges the importance of honor among the warriors of Japan.

Koma hiki toge

A Hokkaido horse trader is rough and earthy by temperament. Nothing bothers him - be it wind, storm, fights, liquor or women - except with his own little daughter, his heart melts.

Komori
(A Baby Sitter)

In farming localities of Japan, many young girls are hired out as baby sitters to help with the family's finances. This sitter tells the baby who is strapped to her back "when you grow up to be a young lady, you will have many lovely kimono and marry a handsome man."

Kon ya-no roku

This dance concerns a daughter of a textile-painter in old Japan. The sophisticated yet haughty and self-centered girl loves to show-off. During one of her dances, she discovers her hands are stained with color and in vain tries to remove the stains with her handkerchief. Although she fails, she continues her performance.

Kora kon, kora kon

Kora kon, kora kon is the sound of Japanese wooden clogs on the street. A girl hears the sound and anticipates a visitor, but the sound fades away.

Kotobuki ondo
Kotobuki ondo is a congratulatory dance.

Kotobuki sanbaso
A ceremonial dance performed for good luck during kabuki dramas.

Kuroda bushi
(Dance of a Samurai)

A samurai from Kuroda in the province of Fukuoka loses his lance to the enemy in battle. He crosses the enemy line to recover his lance and is captured. However, he conducts himself so courageously that the enemy returns the lance to him.

Kurokami
(Raven Hair)

A raven-haired mistress with the help of her little maid is in her boudoir trying on her kimono and enjoying a smoke. The little maid soon tires and becomes sleepy and her mistress scolds her. The dance closes with the mistress dressing the little girl in one of the beautiful kimono.

Kushimoto bushi
(A Folk Dance of Fishermen)

In many Japanese dances, the fan and parasol are the standard props. In this number towels symbolize the valued aspects of the life of the fishermen in Wakayama--the rowing of boats--the rolling of the waves--the casting of nets and other actions connected with fishing and with the sea are part of this dance.

Kutsu ga naru
(The Jingle of the Bells on Our Shoes)

The little girls with their hands joined are playing in the meadow lane. They hop like little rabbits and sing like tiny birds and all the while the bells on their shoes jingle merrily.

Kyoto ningyo
(Kyoto Dolls)

This is the story of some Japanese dolls from the city of Kyoto. They have been sold and must go to Tokyo. To leave their beautiful city of Kyoto and to part with all their dear friends make the dolls very, very sad.

Maiko
(Apprentice Geisha)

A maiko is an apprentice geisha. Her training consists of singing, dancing and impeccable etiquette. In this number, the little maiko gracefully uses parasols and fans. The lovely Kyoto scenery is in the background and the girls are inspired by the beautiful mountains in the distance and the pale moon above.

Maisugata
(Portrait of a Dancing Maiden)

A beautiful dancing maiden is giving up all her personal desires, and even love, to master the art of dancing.

Makina no sanosa

Geisha are dancing to a song which tells of their loves and their heartaches their lovers bring them.

Mari to tono sama

This is a children's dance about a game of ball bouncing. As these little girls are playing the ball bounces away and falls into a lord's treasure box. The box with the ball inside is taken to the lord's castle and the children do not see it again.

Masatsura

Based on a historical event, this story tells of a young warrior of nine who accompanies his father out into the battlefield. Because the boy is too young, the father sends his son home with instructions to always maintain his loyalty to the Emperor. Riding homeward on his horse, Masatsura falls asleep and dreams that his father is killed in the campaign. The dream proves to be true. Remembering his father's advice the boy grows up to become Japan's symbol of courage and loyalty.

Masurao

This is a historic recounting of the fate of nineteen young samurai--warriors--who fought bravely under their provincial lord. Their army has been defeated and the code of the warrior dictates that these nineteen survivors must commit suicide so as not to become captives. These are very young warriors -twelve to fifteen years of age. They accept their fate calmly and their last and only wish is that their parents know that their sons were courageous to the end.

Matsu no miodori

This is a very stylized ceremonial dance which is performed as the opening number of many kabuki dramas. This dance is based on the symbol of the pine tree which denotes long life and endurance.

Matsuri zake
(Festivals of Tokyo)

During the course of the year, people in Tokyo have many festivals to celebrate. A young girl sips rice wine during one of the festivals and romantic experiences of her lost love come back to haunt her.

Matsu zukushi
(Many Shapes of the Pine Tree)

This is a dance that denotes good luck and good cheer. In Japan, the pine tree is held in great esteem because it symbolizes strength and endurance. With the use of fans, these dancers form 10 different shapes of a pine tree. For example, a gracefully shaped tree by a pond, a misshapen pine on a cliff, a lone pine in a rock garden. This is a very difficult number in the traditional style.

Meiji ichidai onna
(Girl of the Meiji Era)

Meiji ichidai onna is a woman who exemplifies the spirit of the Meiji era. She gives up her own career to help the man she loves achieve his ambition.

Meiso nippongo

Nippongo is the name of a famous lance of an equally famous warrior of old Japan. This warrior loses his lance in battle, crosses the enemy lines to retrieve it, is caught and brought before the leader. So bravely and nobly does he conduct himself that out of admiration, the enemy returns his lance.

Men odori

A comic dance with masks that depicts the eternal love triangle.

Mitsumen komori
(A Babysitter in Three Masks)

This is the story of a love triangle between two men and a woman that a baby sitter uses to entertain the children.

Mizu gei
(Water Fantasy)

This is a summer specialty dance. The performer stages a water show suggesting the many forms that can be made with water--for example, a fountain, a waterfall and a misty spray.

Momiji no hashi

Equal in beauty to the cherry blossoms in springtime in Japan are the flaming red and bright yellow maple trees in the autumn. This dance is a classical dance that uses the autumnal theme of the beautiful maple trees.

Musume byakko tai

This dance is based on a story about a historical battle fought by dedicated young warriors. Women also joined in the battle. One young girl carries her injured sister away from the fighting and after witnessing her death commits suicide.

Musume dojoji
(The Lady of the Bell)

In this story taken from a kabuki drama, a beautiful girl is madly in love with a priest. She pursues him relentlessly, but since he cannot return her love, he hides underneath the temple bell. The girl's hate and anger turns her into a serpent. The serpent then wraps itself seven times around the temple bell. The children in this number are the novices who pray for the soul of the dancer so that she might be reborn into a better life.

Musume jinji

This dance tells the plight of a female gambler. Because of her shameful occupation, she cannot go home but is destined to wander from pillar to post. Because she lives in constant danger, she has become skillful with the sword.

Nakanori-san

Nakanori is the name of a Shrine in the central mountains of Japan. This is an old folk dance of these mountain people.

Nan kai no bi sho nen
(A Young Martyr of the South Seas)

In the middle of the 17th century, there was a time when Christians were persecuted by the Tokugawa government. This is the story of a young man who fought and died for his faith.

Nangoku tosa o ato ni shite
(Fond Memories of Tosa)

This song was a very popular pop tune in Japan some years ago. The dancers perform a modern number which popularizes the locale of Tosa.

Naragawa enka

Romantic love ballad of the Naragawa River in the Gifu Prefecture.

Natsu no odori
(A Summer's Dance)

This is a traditional summer odori celebrating the Tanabata festival which falls on the 7th day of the 7th month. Tanabata festival is based upon an ancient legend. On this evening the weaver Princess Star is said to meet the Herd Boy Star on the banks of the River of Heaven for their annual tryst.

Ningyo

My favorite doll. A little girl is playing with her favorite doll. It is hard for her to decide which kimono and which geta or wooden shoes she should put on her doll. She also pretends that the doll is crying and tries to put her to sleep.

Ninin dojoji

There are two girls at Dojoji temple.

Nippon kodomo matsuri

This celebration in honor of children falls in autumn. Following the beating drums, the children go to shrines to offer prayers of thanksgiving.

Nozaki kouta

The little ballad is based on a legend of Nozaki that if you pay a respect to the shrine your "love wish" will come true.

Ochiudo
(The Story of Okaru and Kampei)

This dance is based on a historical story. Okaru and Kampei are lovers in the service of a lord's household. Strict regulations forbid them from expressing their personal feelings. The lord's wife, realizing the situation, persuades the couple to return home to their parents. On their journey home, the two learn that the lord has been forced to commit suicide according to the traditional code of honor. Kampei feeling guilty for failing his master decides also to commit suicide, but Okaru persuades him to go to her home and wait for an opportunity to avenge their lord's disgrace. At this point, Bonnai, a comic figure bursts upon them, attempting to take the girl. This villain attacks Kampei mistaking him for an easy conquest. But Kampei overcomes the villain and escapes.

Oedo nihonbashi

This is the dance about a famous bridge in Tokyo during the turn of the century. The dancers tells the story of the bustling scene on and near the bridge.

Ogi no mato
(The Marksman's Target)

A samurai who is a skilled archer is commanded by his general to shoot a challenging target. The target is being tossed over the ocean on very rough waves. He skillfully hits the bulls eye much to the admiration of all.

Ohana han

Ohana han is the main character of a TV soap opera in Japan. Having lost her husband in the war she is struggling to raise her children alone. Her cheerful disposition and outgoing nature help to ease many of the day to day problems that she must face.

Ohara bushi

This number is a folk dance from the island of Kyushu. The words are in the Kyushu dialect and the movements show the many sides of life on this island.

Oharame
(The Ohara Girl)

The pretty girls of Ohara, a mountain town north of Kyoto, used to commute daily to the city to sell fire wood. This piece is a parody of the popular dance motif of the woman who suffers because of unrequited love. part of the challenge and appeal of "The Ohara Girl" is the dancer's playing both the girl and the man who loves her.

Okichi Monogatari
(The Story of Okichi)

The story of Okichi's effort to save her lover by returning an important sword to him.

Oiwake gasa
(Vagabond)

This dance tells the story of a gambler. He has no permanent home but must go where fortune beckons. Because he is at the mercy of lady luck, he can never fall in love.

Okesa chidori
(Sandpiper Dance)

A geisha, watching the sandpipers flitting along the beach, longs sentimentally for her lover.

Okesa kuzushi

A typical Japanese folk dance based on a folk song of the Niigata prefecture.

Okichi monogatari
(Story of Okichi)

This is a buyo rendition of the kabuki piece based on the bunraku puppet drama of the story of Okichi.

Okosa de nunoko

This is a comic folk dance of the farming region of Akita. Social situations of a boy-girl relationships are enacted. One scene tells of a girl being stood up. She cooked a meal of noodles for her boyfriend and she waits for his rival but he fails to appear.

Omiwa
(Name of a Maiden)

This dance is taken from a kabuki play about a triangle love affair between: a maiden, a princess, and a samurai.

Omoide zake

A hostess is drinking sake by herself thinking of a parted lover. She wishes that one day he will return to her. This is a popular modern ballad.

Omokage zakura

The famous Tokyo shrine called Yasukuni Jinga is a war memorial to Japanese soldiers who died in the war. A mother dances at the shrine in memory of her son who was a soldier. She recalls the day her son went off to war and how bravely she sent him off.

Onatsu kyoran
(Lovesick Onatsu)

An introduction to a new style kabuki. Onatsu is gradually losing her mind over her concern for her lover who is sent to prison. She sees his image as she walks down a country road and is taunted by the children.

Onatsu seijiro
(Romantic Dance)

A very famous story is told in this dance. A wealthy rice dealer's daughter Onatsu falls in love with her father's clerk, Seijiro. Because they are of different social standing and can never marry they elope. As they are about to escape in a boat, they are caught. The girl must go back to her parents and her lover is sent to prison for stealing money from the rice business.

Orite yuku
(A Geisha Dance)

Orite yuku is a geisha dance depicting the reflections of a professional entertainer who longs for quiet and solitude.

Osaka zuki
(A Cup of Rice Wine)

This is taken from a famous historical story telling of a courageous samurai, a feudal warrior. He has come into the enemy, he is invited to drink wine and to dance. He conducts himself so honorably that he is highly praised and is given back his lance.

Osaru no kagoya
(The Monkey's Carriage)

Two little monkeys are organized into a taxi-cab business. Their taxi, however, does not have wheels, but must be carried litter-fashion on their shoulders. The little monkeys do get terribly tired and hot, but their carriage is very convenient because it can go over rocks, under fences, just about anywhere that you can imagine.

Osho
(The Champion Chess Player)

This dance tells the feelings of a shogi player. Shogi is a Japanese board game resembling chess. The dance dramatizes his burning desire to win the championship tournament.

Osome kyoran: Osome and Hisanatsu

This is a famous dance taken from kabuki plays. It is a beautiful love story about two teen age lovers who prepare to die.

Otemoyan
(Comical Dance)

This dance is a comic dance with the words in the dialect of the province of Kumamoto. The woman says, "I went to get married, but I did not like my husband-to-be's face. But I suppose my go-betweens will arrange something else for me. You know, I came to see you because even though you're not terribly handsome, I like the beautiful gold cigarette box you carry there in your hip pocket."

Otoko de yoisho

A man with true grit has only himself on which to depend. He does what he must do and if he fails, he has only himself to blame. The words of the song tell us that if a man were to stumble seven times, the eighth time he would get up and start anew. Determination and courage are the measure of a man.

Otoko nara
(If I Were a Man)

This dance enacts the wishes of a girl. She thinks: If I were a man, I would wear the formal attire of a samurai--a warrior. I would put on the hakama and crested kimono and I would go to war and bravely defend my lord. A sash ties the kimono so movement is freer and a hachimaki, or head band helps to generate physical strength.

Otoko no shiro

This is in praise of the beautiful feudal castle of Matsuyama on the island of Shikoku. Built on the shores of the Island Sea, it stands proud and stately due to its excellence in design of a famous architect, Kato Yoshioki.

Otome tsubaki

The tsubaki is the lovely camellia. On Oshima an island in Tokyo Bay, the camellia blooms in profusion. This song tells a story of a young lady who goes down to the seashore to fetch water and at the water's edge gazes out across the sea in the direction of her loved one who has sailed away.

Otsuki sama
(Mr. Moon)

The moon centers as the theme of many Japanese songs and dances. This dance tells how youthful the moon looks year after year. It never grows old although it does change. When it is crescent shaped, it resembles the arched eyebrows of my beautiful sister. And when it is full, it resembles the lovely bouffant hair style of a beautiful maiden.

Ozashiki kouta
(Dance of Geisha)

The dance of two young women studying to be geisha.

Pyon pyokorin

In this dance two little white rabbits dance and cavort as they wait for their mother to come.

Reiho fuji

This dance tells of the beautiful symmetry of mount Fuji. Because of its near perfect cone shape, this mountain is held sacred by the Japanese people.

Renjishi
(The Lions)

This is the story of a lion king who is training its cub to be fearless and strong. The lion throws the cub down a steep cliff and watches it climb to the top. But as soon as it does, the lion kicks it down again. This is repeated many times, but each time, the cub claws its way to the top. Finally, the father is satisfied that his son has the strength and heart to be a true king of beasts. They both rejoice and the dance ends on a joyous note.

Ribon no yume
(Dream of Ribbons)

A lovely child falls asleep with a beautiful ribbon in her hair. In her dreams, she sees the ribbon become a butterfly fluttering in the breeze in the clear, blue sky. She awakens to find that she has fallen asleep with bells in her long kimono sleeves.

Ringo no hitori goto

This dance tells of apples picked from the orchard on the train to the city markets. The apples are longing to be back in the orchards, wandering about the old farmer and his work.

Rokudan
(Dance in Six Parts)

The training of a young lady born of high social standing is intensive. To attain the social graces, she must study the art of tea ceremony, flower arrangement, calligraphy, odori and music. This dance is very stylized in the manner of the classical odori.

Rokudan kuzushi

This is one of the many folk dances that are traditionally popular in Japan. These dancers perform with fans in the odori.

Sado okesa

A folk song from the island of Sado. There are many legends as to the origin of the word Okesa. One legend goes--Once upon a time, a rich old man lived on the isle. Eventually he went broke and he only had a cat which he loved dearly. The cat felt sorry for the poor master and transformed itself into a beautiful geisha girl, calling herself Okesa. Okesa's singing and dancing earned much fame and riches for her. Her dance and song became known as Okesa.

Sagi musume
(The Spirit of the Snow Heron)

It was the day of the long awaited marriage of the young couple in love. As the bridal procession came to the side of the pond, a masked man broke into the procession and killed the bride. This man was a young samurai whose sweetheart was being forced to marry another man on this same day. In despair, he planned to kill his sweetheart and commit suicide. As he looked at the girl who lay before him, he realizes that he killed the wrong girl. Since that tragic day, a beautiful snow heron has made her home by the pond and can be seen dancing all alone. The villagers claim that this is the spirit of the unfortunate girl reliving the happy days of the past.

Saitoro bushi
(The Boatmen's Dance)

This dance has a very pronounced beat almost like the beat of Indian drums. This song is sung when the fishermen from Miyagi go out to sea and when they heavy nets filled with their catch are hauled aboard the boats. The rhythm provides the cadence to which these men work.

Sakura kamuro
(Cherry Blossoms Maidens)

Two little maids-in-waiting to a consort go on an errand carrying letters. On the way, they play under the cherry trees, scattering petals and making bouncing balls out of the blossoms.

Sakura rokudan

The melody of this composition is taken from a classical composition. Rokudan is a dance in six parts. The dancers are admiring the spring landscape of lovely cherry blossoms.

Sankatsu hanhichi

Osono, the dancer in this number is a very tragic figure. Her marriage to Hanhichi has been arranged by the two families is not a love match. Hanhichi has a courtesan as his true love. To support the courtesan and their child, Hanhichi embezzles money. Although he has brought disgrace upon the family, Osono refuses to divorce him, believing that it is her duty to stay with her husband. This dance shows her at home in great anxiety wondering if her husband will return. As she waits, many thoughts pass through her mind. She has resolved that even if her impossible situation means committing suicide, she will not leave her husband and return to her parents. When thoughts of suicide cross the dancer's mind, she draws forth a razor which is designed for women to slit their throats.

Sanosa
A Kyoto geisha is dancing and singing of her love for her patron. Her love for him has grown gradually over the years and now she is anxiously awaiting to see him again.

Sanosa bushi
Coming home from her evening's work and a little intoxicated from the sake she has drunk, the professional entertainer strolls along thinking of her true love. It is her lot to be a dancing girl but she cannot help thinking and wandering about him.

Sanosa kuzushi
This number is a variation of an old song entitled "Sanosa." Similar to our nostalgic mood, Japan has revived a number of the old goodies.

Sansa shigure
This folk song comes from the island of Kyushu. This is the battle song sung by the local people to raise the spirits of the warriors who are going to battle.

Sarashime
Japanese silk with its brilliantly dyed colors is world famous. In this dance the setting is one of the eight famous scenic sites of Omi located near Kyoto which is famous for its dye works. The young maidens, dyers, are rinsing and bleaching the dye materials in a stream. The movement of the banner represents the swift flowing waters of the stream.

Sei kai ha
This song is of the three most beautiful scenic spots in Japan: Matsushima, Amano Hashidate and Miyajima.

Seki no go hon machi

Pine trees in Japan are a symbol of constancy and devotion. This dance concerns a prehistoric deity of five pine trees planted on a mound. Because of the uneven number a great lord wants one of these five trees to be cut down. After many centuries of controversy, the five trees are still standing near this scenic ocean spot.

Sekirei no mai
(Dance of a Pair of Birds)

Sekirei no mai depicts a love story danced by a pair of birds. They display a deep happiness in meeting again after a long period of being apart.

Shami de odori

This is a geisha dance. A geisha is telling her customer that they can try a western style dance with shamisen.

Shichi go san

This translated means seven, three and five. There is a belief in Japan that children of the ages of three, five, and seven are the most vulnerable to sickness and in the November festival the dancers plead to the spirits to protect the children of these age groups. The children receive toys and sweetmeats on this occasion.

Shikararete
(A Baby Sitter's song)

In farming localities in Japan, young girls are often hired out as baby sitters. This story tells of a young baby sitter who works for a family far from her home. Sent on an errand at dusk, she becomes frightened in the dark and cries for the comfort of her mother's arms. In a few months spring will come--but will she be home to see the lovely wild flowers.

Shima no burusu
(Blues of Shima)

This is a popular song from the island of Okinawa. A historic site which figured so prominently in World War II. Western influences can be seen in the dance forms. There is much more movement of the hips than in the classical odori and the foot placement is in the style of western ballet.

Shima sodachi

This is an Okinawa song telling of a lovely girl born and raised on one of these islands. The girls from this locale are known for their beautiful raven hair. The dancers interpret by their movements the deep longing they have for their loved ones who have sailed away from these islands.

Shinganoko
(Dancing Maidens)

Beautiful maidens clad in colorful kanako or kimono dance to recreate the character of Shirabyoshi, a famous dancer from a kabuki drama. The many moods and expressions of this famous dancer are interpreted by the graceful movements of our performers.

Shinyoku ura shima

Traditionally, all kabuki dances and dramas are opened with a very stylized type of ceremonial number. The Japanese believe that this type of opening number will clear the air of evil so the good luck will prevail throughout the evening. The dance is based on the symbol of the ocean waves which denote everlasting strength.

Shiokumi
(Dipping the Brine)

This dance derives from the noh play "Matsukaze" (Pine Wind) about a girl salt maker named Matsukaze, who was loved and abandoned by a handsome courtier in exile. She enters wearing the court robe he left her, and carries her salt buckets. "Shiokumi" is a challenging piece because the dancer must express Matsukaze's many different moods--nostalgia, longing, loneliness, and anticipation--and she must hand difficult stage properties with skill and grace.

Shirasagi no shiro
(White Heron Castle)

There is a very sad story connected with the white heron castle in Himeji, Hyogo. During the feudal days, a beautiful princess was forced into a marriage and came to live in this castle. On the wall of one of the rooms in which she spent many unhappy hours, there is painted a masterpiece of a white heron. In this number, the performers are feudal warriors enacting this tragic story.

Shishi no rankyoku
A dance which shows a father lion throwing his son into a ravine to test his strength and courage. At the end of the test he celebrates his son's triumph over his fears.

Shitadashi sanbaso
Classical ceremonial number often performed as opening number at kabuki program.

Shochikubai
(Pine, Bamboo, and Plum)
These are the three felicitous plants and "Shochikubai" is a celebratory dance to open the show. Pine is prized for its longevity, bamboo for its pliancy, plum for its blossoming despite cold winds and snow. The lyrics combine pine, bamboo, and plum imagery with joyful scenes from Japan's major holiday celebrations. The piece can be done my many dancers.

Sho genroki bayashi
This lively song tells of modern Japan, a Japan that is enjoying prosperity and an excitement that it has never known before.

Sho sama mairu
This is a traditional comic story of Fukushima. A girl working out as a maid writes a letter to her boyfriend back in her village. In comic fashion, she gives him all sorts of advice on his conduct.

Sho shojoji
(In the Garden of the Shojo Temple)
The badger plays a large role in Japanese folklore. He has the power to cast spells on people and trick them in many situations. In this dance, the badger is dancing in the gardens of Shojo temple. It is a beautiful moonlit night and this creature prances about thumping his popped stomach like a drum.

Showa sanosa
This is a song written at the turn of the century and rearranged during the Showa period. It considers the work of an artist Umegi Yaka Ni Sa and the poses of his model who is in a traditional kimono costume, but creates effects that are modern.

Sooshi

Sooshi means spun thread and is a symbol of a human life. Shizuka Gozen, the wife of Yoritomo, a military governor goes into exile when her husband is defeated. Her dance enacts the hard life she must endure in her exile.

Soran bushi

A folk song from the island of Hakkaido. This song is sung by the fishermen while they are pulling in their catch. It is so named from the shouting to mark time like Yo Yo or Heave Ho. The fishermen have to draw in their nets all together in good rhythm, since the herring come in schools large enough to change the color of the sea.

Suehiro gari
(Interpretation of the Fan)

A folding fan is called suehiro, a symbol of expanding good luck and happiness, and is used on auspicious occasions. A daimyo and her servant perform this dance taken from medieval drama.

Suma no yugure
(Evening Scenes of Suma)

This is a dance of the beauty of the area around Suma.

Taketori monogatari
(Wood cutter's tale)

This is the story of a woodcutter.

Taki no shiraito
(A Taisho Ballad)

This is a song written during the Taisho period. A traveling female musician is in love with a poor student and personally goes into debt to pay a loan shark. Ultimately, the student becomes a judge and the performer who helped him financially is brought before him for dealing with illicit money lenders. However, she is happy because of the former lover's success.

Tamaya
(The Bubble Vender)

In the Edo period there were many types of street vendors selling various items. Two of these vendors were a soap bubble vender and a butterfly vender.

These vendors illustrate, with light movements, the mood and lives of the people during the Edo period.

Tanko bushi
(Coal Miner's Dance)
This is a folk dance portraying the work of the coal miner.

Tawara tsumi uta
This dance depicts a farmer celebrating a rice harvest, stacking bales of rice into storage. The song is from the Amori prefecture.

Tobi ume no fu
(Essence of the Plum Blossoms)
This is a historical dance about the temple maids dancing for their court noble and pretending to be plum blossoms.

Toribe yama shinjyu
(Lover's Suicide on Mt. Toribe)
A geisha and her lover who have committed murder are running away to Mt. Toribe, a famous mountain noted for love suicides.

Tsugaru jongara bushi
(A Rhythmic Tune from Tsugaru)
This is a folk dance that features the use of many fans.

Ukiyo dojoji
This is a variant of the famous Dojoji story of a woman so angry at being betrayed in love that she becomes a demon incarnate. In "Ukiyo dojoji" the dancer plays a courtesan longing for her lover. The tolling of the Dojoji temple bell tells her that he is leaving.

Yagiri no watashi
This was the most popular ballad of 1983 in Japan. The theme is the elopement of two lovers whose parents do not approve of their relationship.

Yagura ondo
This is a summer festival folk dance using the drum for a heavy beat and like other ondo contains a repetition of simple dance steps and hand movements. An audience could participate with very little instruction.

Yakko-san
(Lord's Little Helpers)
The children help the lord of a feudal castle.

Yakkuken
(Baseball Dance)
A dance depicting the movements from baseball.

Yanagi no ame
(Willow in the Rain)
This is a classical selection. A young musician is walking in the rain, as she is playing her instrument she is remembering the camellia flowers. The willows wet with rain look to her as if they are crying.

Yosaku
(Mr. Yosaku)
This has been a popular Japanese song. Mr. Yosaku is a timber toper. His wife is calling for him as he chops trees in the forest. He compliments his wife who is busy weaving from early morn till late at night.

Yoshiwara suzume
(The Bird Vendors of Yoshiwara)
A man and his wife selling sparrows describe in their dance the beautiful scenery and the daily life of the women in the Yoshiwara entertainment district.

Yuname chidori
(Dance of the Plover)
In the quiet of the evening, the sad cries of the plover are heard as they fly over the waves along the beach.

Yuzuki sendo
(Excursion)
Boat men under the evening moon.

Yuzuru no mai
(Dance of the Cranes at Sunset)
The dancer in this dance depicts the dances of the cranes at sunset.

APPENDIX B

THE TEN MOST TAUGHT DANCES IN EACH AGE CATEGORY

CHILDREN (5-12)	TEEN-AGERS (12-18)	ADULTS (18 and over)
Ehi gasa (The Parasol Dance)	Aki no irokusa (The Colored Grasses of Autumn)	Ame no goro (The Revenge of Goro)
Hanakage (Beneath the Flowers)	Chakkiri bushi (Women of the Tea Leaves)	Fuji musume (Wisteria Maiden)
Kasabutai (Dance in two parts)	Echigo jishi (Lion Dancer of Echigo)	Harusame (Spring Rain)
Kawaii sakanaya san (A Little Fish Vendor)	Genroku hanami odori (Cherry Blossom Dance)	Kotobuki sanbaso (Sanbaso Piece)
Kikuzukushi (Chrysanthemum Dance)	Harusame jishi (A Lion Dancer in the Spring Rain)	Kurokami (Raven Hair)
Maiko (Dancing Girl)	Itsuki no komori ningyo (The Baby sitter Doll)	Mitsumen komori (A baby sitter in three masks)
Maisugata (Portrait of a Dancing Maiden)	Kocho no mai (Dance of the Butterflies)	Musume dojoji (Lady of the Bell)
Ningyo (A Doll)	Soran bushi (Fish Harvesting Song)	Oharame (The Ohara Girl)
Otsuki sama (Mr. Moon)	Tobi ume no fu (Spirit of the Plum Blossoms)	Taki no shiraito (A Taisho Ballad)
Sakura kamuro (Cherry Blossom Maidens)	Yuname chidori (Dance of the Plover)	Yoshiwara suzume (Bird Vender of Yoshiwara)

REFERENCES

Agar, M. 1980. *The Professional Stranger*. New York: Academic Press.
Araki, J. T. 1964. *The Ballad Drama of Medieval Japan*. Los Angeles: University of California Press.
Arnott, P. 1969. *The Theaters of Japan*. London: MacMillan.
Ashihara, E. 1964. *The Japanese Dance*. Tokyo: Japan Travel Bureau.
Baldwin, L. 1989, August 12. Japanese dancers shine in riveting show. *The Spokesman Review*, p. 4.
Barnland, D. 1975. *Public and Private Self in Japan and the United States*. Tokyo: Simul Press.
Barba, E. 1982. Theatre anthropology. *Drama Review* 94:5-32.
Barth, F. 1969. *Ethnic Groups and Boundaries*. Boston: Little Brown.
Bertaux, D., (Ed.). 1981. *Biography and Society*. California: SAGE.
Bethe, M., & Brazell, K. 1990. The practice of noh theatre. In Schechner, R. & Appel, L. (Eds.). *By Means of Performance* (167-193). New York: Cambridge University Press.
Birdwhistell, R. 1970. *Kinesics and Context*. Philadelphia: University of Pennsylvania Press.
Blacker, C. 1975. *The Catalpa Bow*. London: Allen & Unwin.
Blacking, J. 1977. *Towards an Anthropology of the Body*. London: Academic Press.
Bowers, F. 1952. *Japanese Theater*. New York: Hermitage House.

Bowers, F. 1956. *Theater in the East: A Survey of Asian Dance and Drama*. New York: Grove Press.
Brandon, J., Malm, W., & Shively, D. 1978. *Studies in Kabuki*. Honolulu: University of Hawaii Press.
Brandon, J. 1978. Training at the Waseda Little Theatre. *Drama Review* 22:29-42.
Brandon, J. 1989. Asian theatre in the west today. *Drama Review* 33:25-50.
Burgess, M. E. 1978. The resurgence of ethnicity: Myth or reality. *Ethnic and Racial Studies* 1:265-285.
Buruma, I. 1984. *Behind the Mask*. New York: Panthenon Books.
Castile, G. P., & Kushner, G. (Ed.). 1981. *Persistent Peoples*. Arizona: University of Arizona Press.
Chai, A. Y. 1988. Women's history in public: picture brides of Hawaii. *Women's Studies Quarterly* 1: 51-62.
Clifford, J. 1988. *The Predicament of Culture*. Cambridge: Harvard University Press.
Clifford, J., & Marcus, G. (Eds.). 1986. *Writing Culture*. Los Angeles: University of California Press.
Coaldrake, K. 1989. Female Tayu in the Gidayu narrative tradition of Japan. In Koskoff, E. (Ed.). *Women in Music in Cross-cultural Perspective* (pp. 151-163). Chicago: University of Illinois Press.
Cohen, S. J., & Maksakastsu, G. 1983. Virtuosity and the aesthetic ideals of Japanese dance and virtuosity and the aesthetic ideals of western classical dance. *Dance Research Journal* 14:88-97.
Collier, M. J., & Thomas, M. 1988. Cultural identity: An interpretive perspective. In Kim, Y. Y. (Ed.). *Theories in Intercultural Communication* (pp. 99-120). London: SAGE.
Conroy, H., & Miyakawa, T. (Eds.). 1972. *East Across the Pacific*. Oxford, England: American Bibliographical Center.
Coombs, J. 1981. The O'bon festival in Los Angeles. Unpublished manuscript.
Crapanzano, V. 1980. *Tuhami: Portrait of a Moroccan*. Chicago: University of Chicago Press.
Dalby, L. 1983. *Geisha*. Berkeley: University of California Press.
Daniels, R. 1990. *Coming to America*. New York: Harper Collins.
Davis, M. (Ed.) 1982. *Interaction Rhythms*. New York: Human Sciences Press.
Despres, L. 1978. Toward a theory of ethnic phenomena. In Despres, L. (Ed.). *Ethnicity and Resource Competition in Plural Societies*. (pp. 187-107). The Hague: Mouton.

De Vos, G. (Ed.). 1976. *Responses to Change: Society, Culture and Personality.* New York: D. Van Nostrand.
De Vos, G., & Romanucci-Ross, L. (Eds.). 1982. *Ethnic Identity.* Chicago: University of Chicago Press.
Douglas, J. 1985. *Creative Interviewing.* London: SAGE.
Dunn, C., & Torigoe, B. 1969. *The Actor's Analects.* Tokyo: University of Tokyo Press.
Eaton, A. H. 1952. *Beauty Behind Barbed Wire.* New York: Harper Brothers.
Erikson, E. 1959. *Identity and the Life Cycle.* New York: International Universities.
Erikson, E. 1968. *Identity Youth and Crisis.* New York: W.W. Norton.
Erickson, E. 1975. *Life History and the Historical Moment.* New York: Norton.
Ernst, E. 1974. *The Kabuki Theatre.* Honolulu: University of Hawaii Press.
Fukei, B. 1976. *The Japanese American Story.* Minneapolis, Minnesota: Dillion Press.
Gans, H. J. 1979. Symbolic anthropology: The future of ethnic groups and cultures in America. *Ethnic and Racial Studies* 2:1-20.
Georges, R. A., & Jones, M. 1980. *People Studying People.* Los Angeles: University of California Press.
Glazer, N., & Moynihan, D. (Eds.). 1975. *Ethnicity and Experience.* Cambridge: Harvard University Press.
Glenn, E. 1986. *Issei, Nisei, War Bride: Three Generations of Japanese-Americans in Domestic Service.* New York: Temple University Press.
Golde, P. (Ed.). 1970. *Women in the Field.* Chicago: Aldine.
Gottschalk, L. 1947. *Use of Personal Documents in History.* Michigan: Edwards Brothers.
Greely, A. 1974. *Ethnicity in the United States.* New York: Wiley.
Gudykunst, K., Kim, Y. Y. (Eds.). 1988. *Theories in Intercultural Communication.* Beverly Hills: SAGE.
Gunji, M. 1970. *Buyo.* New York, Tokyo, and Kyoto: Weatherhill/Tankosha.
Gunji, M. 1985. *Kabuki.* Tokyo and Palo Alto: Kondansha International.
Halford, A. S., & Giovanna, M. 1971. *The Kabuki Handbook.* Rutland, Vermont: Charles E. Tuttle.
Hall, E. 1969. *The Hidden Dimension.* New York: Anchor Books.
Hall, E. 1977. *Beyond Culture.* New York: Anchor Books.
Hanamura, Y. 1956. *Kabuki.* (Fume Takano, Trans.). Tokyo: Kenkyusha.
Hanna, J. L. 1988. *Dance, Sex and Gender.* Chicago: University of Chicago Press.

Haseltine, P. 1989. *East and Southeast Asian Material Culture in North America*. New York: Greenwood Press.
Havens, T. 1982. *Artist and Patron in Postwar Japan*. Princeton: Princeton University Press.
Havens, T. 1983. Rebellion and expression in contemporary Japanese dance. *Dance Research Annual* 14:159-165.
Hendry, J., Weber J. (Eds.). 1986. *Interpreting Japanese Society*. Oxford: JASO.
Henry, F. 1976. *Ethnicity in the Americas*. The Hague: Mouton Publishers.
Hicks, G., & Leis, P. (Eds.). 1977. *Ethnic Encounters*. Massachusetts: Duxbury Press.
Hoff, F. 1983. Dojoji, a woman and a bell. *Dance Research Journal* 14:32-41.
Honda, Y. 1974. Yamabushi Kagura and Bugaku: performance in the Japanese middle ages and contemporary folk performance. (Frank Hoff, Trans.). *Educational Theatre Journal* 26:192-208.
Hosokawa, B. 1969. *Nisei: The Quiet Americans*. New York: William Morrow & Company.
Hsu, F. L. K. 1975. *Iemoto: The Heart of Japan*. New York: John Wiley and Sons.
Ito, K. 1973. *Issei*. Japan: Japan Publications.
Ito, S. 1979. Some characteristics of Japanese expression as they appear in dance. *Dance Research Journal* 12:267-281.
Izutsu, T. and T. 1981. *The Theory of Beauty in the Classical Aesthetics of Japan*. London: Martinus Nijhoff.
Johnson, C. 1974. *The Presentational Style of an Onnagata*. Unpublished Master's Thesis, University of Oregon.
Johnson, M. 1987. *The Body in the Mind*. Chicago: University of Chicago Press.
Juhan, D. 1987. *Job's Body*. Barrytown, New York: Station Hill Press.
Kasho, M. 1969. Japanese music and dance. *Japanese Culture in the Meiji Era*. Tokyo: Heibunsha.
Kato, S. 1979. *A History of Japanese Literature*. Tokyo: Kodansha International.
Kawatake, T. 1971. *Japan on Stage*. Tokyo: 3A Corp.
Keene, D. 1961. *Major Plays of Chikamatsu*. New York: Columbia University Press.
Keene, D. 1973. *Noh: The Classical Theatre of Japan*. New York: Harper & Row.
Keene, D. 1988. *The Pleasures of Japanese Literature*. New York: Columbia University Press.
Kikumura, A. 1981. *Through Harsh Winters*. California: Chandler & Sharp.

Kim, Y. Y. & Ruben, B. D. 1988. Intercultural transformation: A systems theory. In Kim, Y. Y. (Ed.). *Theories in Intercultural Communication* (pp. 299-321). London: SAGE.

Kincaid, J. 1925. *Kabuki: The Popular Stage of Japan.* Toronto: MacMillan.

King, E. 1979. The way of Japanese dance. *Mimes, Mask and Marionette* 2:80-103.

Kirk, J., & Miller, M. 1986. *Reliability and Validity in Qualitative Research.* London: SAGE.

Kitagawa, D. 1967. *Issei and Nisei: The Internment Years.* New York: The Seabury Press.

Kitano, H. L. 1976. *Japanese Americans.* Los Angeles: University of California Press.

Kitano, H. L., & Daniels, R. 1988. *Asian Americans: Emerging Minorities.* New Jersey: Prentice Hall.

Kleinman, S. (Ed.). 1986. *Mind and Body: East Meets West.* Illinois: Human Kinetics Publishers.

Kominz, L. 1983. The genesis of a Kabuki aragoto classic. *Monumenta Nipponica* 38:387-407.

Kominz, L. 1985. The Soga revenge story: Tradition and innovation in Japanese drama. (Doctoral dissertation, Columbia University, 1984). *Dissertation Abstracts*, 46A, 703.

Kozo, Y. 1983. Early Kabuki dance. *Dance Research Journal* 14:105-114.

Kwon, Y. H. K. 1988. The female entertainment tradition in medieval Japan: The case of the Asobi. *Theatre Journal* 40:205-216.

Langness, L. L., & Frank, G. 1981. *Lives: An Anthropological Approach to Biography.* California: Chandler & Sharp.

Lebra, T. S. 1976. *Japanese Patterns of Behavior.* Honolulu: University of Hawaii Press.

Leiter, S. 1979. *The Art of Kabuki.* Berkeley: University of California Press.

MacAloon, J. J. 1984. *Rite, drama, Festival, Spectacle: Rehearsals Toward a Theory of Cultural Performance.* Philadelpia: Institute for the Study of Human Issues.

Malm, J. R. 1977. The legacy of Nihon Buyo. *Dance Research Journal* 9:12-24.

Malm, J. R. 1985. The meaning of iemoto seido in the world of Nihon Buyo. *Dance Research Journal* 15: 160-171.

Malm, W. 1978. Music in the Kabuki theatre. In Brandon, J., Shively, D. & Malm, W. (Eds.). *Studies in Kabuki* (pp. 133-169). Hawaii: University of Hawaii Press.

Marcus, G. 1986. Contemporary problems of ethnography in the modern world system. In Clifford, J. & Marcus, G. (Eds.). *Writing Culture* (pp. 165-193). Berkeley: University of California Press.
Matida, K. 1938. *Odori*. Japan: Board of Tourist Industry.
Mayo, C., & Henley, N. (Eds.). 1981. *Gender and Nonverbal Behavior*. New York: Springer-Verlag.
McKay, J., & Lewins, F. 1978. Ethnicity and the ethnic group: A conceptual analysis and reformulation. *Ethnic Studies and Racial Studies*, 1:412-27.
McAdams, D. 1985. *Power, Intimacy and the Life Story*. Illinois: Dorsey Press.
Mishler, E. G. 1986. *Research Interviewing*. Cambridge: Harvard University Press.
Miyake, S. 1963. *Kabuki Drama*. Tokyo: Japanese Tourist Bureau.
Morissey, C. 1970. On oral history interviewing. In Dester, L. (Ed.). *Elite and Specialized Interviewing* (pp. 51-70). Evanston: Northwestern University Press.
Munro, T. 1955. *Oriental Aesthetics*. Cleveland, Ohio: Western Reserve University Press.
Murphy, M. 1992. *The Future of the Body*. Los Angeles: Jeremy P. Tarcher.
Nakano, M. T. 1990. *Japanese American Women*. Berkeley: Mina Press Publishing.
Nomura, G. M. 1987. Tsugiki, a grafting: a history of a Japanese pioneer woman in Washington State. *Women's Studies* 15-37.
Novak, M. 1971. *The Rise of the Unmeltable Ethnics*. New York: Macmillan.
O'Brien, D. & Fugita, S. 1991. *The Japanese American Experience*. Bloomington: Indiana University Press.
Okimoto, D. L. 1977. *American in Disguise*. New York: Weatherhill.
Ortner, S. 1979. On key symbols. In Lessa W. & Vogt E. (Eds.). *Reader in Comparative Religion* (pp. 92-98). New York: Harper and Row.
Petersen, W. 1981. *Japanese Americans: Oppression and Success*. Washington D. C.: University Press.
Philippi, D. L. (Trans.). 1969. *Kojiki*. Tokyo: Princeton University Press & Tokyo Press.
Plummer, K. 1983. *Documents of Life*. London: George Allen & Unwin.
Pronko, L. 1967. *Theater East and West: Perspectives Toward a Total theater*. Berkeley, California: University of California Press.
Pronko, L. 1985. Shin Buyo and Sosaku Buyo: Tradition and change in Japanese dance, *Dance Research Annual* 15:111-121.

Ramsey, S. 1984. Double vision: Nonverbal behavior east and west. In Wolfgang, A. (Ed.). *Nonverbal Behavior* (pp. 70-85). Toronto: C. J. Hogrefe.

Raz, J. 1983. *Audience and Actors: A study of their Interaction in the Japanese Traditional Theatre*. Leiden, The Netherlands: E. J. Brill.

Reischauer, E. O. 1981. *The Japanese*. Cambridge: Harvard University Press.

Reminick, R. A. 1983. *Theory of Ethnicity*. New York: University Press of America.

Rimer, T., & Masakazu, Y. 1984. *On the Art of the Noh drama*. Princeton, New Jersey: Princeton University Press.

Rosaldo, R. 1986. From the door of his tent: The fieldworker and the inquistor. In Clifford, J. & Marcus, G. (Eds.). *Writing Culture* (pp 77-97). Berkley: University of California Press.

Royce, A. P. 1977. *The Anthropology of Dance*. Bloomington: University Press.

Royce, A. P. 1982. *Ethnic Identity*. Bloomington: Indiana University Press.

Said, E. 1978. *Orientalism*. New York: Pantheon.

Sarasohn, E. S. (Ed.). 1983. *The Issei: Portrait of a Pioneer*. Palo Alto, California: Pacific Books.

Schechner, R. 1977. *Essays on Performance Theory*. New York: Drama Book Club Specialists.

Schechner, R. 1985. *Between Theatre and Anthropology*. Philadelphia: University of Pennsylvania Press.

Schechner, R., & Appel, W. (Ed). 1990. *By Means of Performance*. New York: Cambridge University Press.

Schmidt, R. 1986. Japanese martial arts as spiritual education. In Kleiman, S. (Ed.). *Mind and Body* (pp. 69-74). Illinois: Human Kinetics.

Scott, A.C. 1955. *The Kabuki Theater of Japan*. London: George Allen.

Seidensticker, E. 1985. *Low City, High City*. San Francisco: Donald S. Ellis.

Sekine, M. 1985. *Ze-ami and his Theories of Noh Drama*. London: Billings & Sons.

Seller, M. (Ed.). 1983. *Ethnic Theatre in the United States*. Connecticut: Greenwood Press.

Shaver, R. M. 1966. *Kabuki Costume*. Rutland, Vermont: Charles Tuttle.

Sheridan, M., & Salaff, J. (Eds.). 1984. *Lives: Chinese Working women*. Bloomington, Indiana: Indiana University Press.

Shigetoshi, K. 1958. *Kabuki: Japanese Drama*. Tokyo, Japan: Foreign Affairs Association of Japan.

Smither, R. 1982. Human migration and the acculturation of minorities. *Human Relations* 35:57-68.
Spicer, E. 1962. *Cycles of Conquest*. Tucson: Univeristy of Arizona.
Spicer, E. 1971. Persistent identity systems. *Science* 4011:795-800.
Stein, H. F., & Hill, R. 1977. *The Ethnic Imperative*. University Park: Pennsylvania State University Press.
Sugiyama, M., & Kanjuro. F. 1937. *An Outline History of the Japanese dance*. Tokyo: Kokusai Bunka Shinkokai.
Suzuki, D. 1959. *Zen and Japanese culture*. Princeton, New Jersey: Princeton University Press.
Takaki, R. 1989. *Strangers from a Different Shore*. London: Penguin Books.
Takashima, S. 1971. *A Child in a Prison Camp*. New York: Mentor.
Tateishi, R. 1969. *Classic Dancing in Japan*. Tokyo: Tokyo Shobo.
Thiele, M. 1987. *Footprints Across Oregon*. Portland, Oregon: Graphic Arts Center.
Toita, Y. 1970. *Kabuki*. New York, Tokyo, and Kyoto: Weatherhill/Tankosha.
Toyotaka, K. 1956. *Japanese Music and Drama in the Meiji Era*. (Donald Keene and Edward Seidensticker, Trans.). Tokyo: Obunsha.
Tsubaki, T. 1971. Zeami and the transition of the concept of yugen. *Journal of Aesthetic and Art Criticism* 30:55-67.
Turner, V. 1982. *From Ritual to Theatre: The Human Seriousness of Play*. New York: Performing Arts Journal Press.
Turner, V. 1986. *The Anthropology of Performance*. New York: Paj.
Ueda, M. 1967. *Literary and Art Theories in Japan*. Cleveland, Ohio: Western Reserve Press.
United States Department of Interior. *People in Motion: the Postwar Adjustment of the Evacuated Japanese Americans*. Washington D. C.: U. S. Goverment Printing Office.
Van Maanen, J. 1988. *Tales of the Field*. Chicago: University of Chicago Press.
Van Zile, J. 1982. *The Japanese Bon dance of Hawaii*. Hawaii: Pacifica Press.
Wagner, J. (Ed.). 1979. *Images of Information*. London: SAGE.
Walls, T. 1987. *The Japanese Texans*. San Antonio, Texas: University of Texas.
Werner, O., & Schoepfle, M. 1987. *Systematic Fieldwork Volumes I and II*. London: SAGE.
Wolfgang, A. (Ed.). 1984. *Nonverbal Behavior*. New York: C. J. Hogrefe.
Yasuji, Honda. 1983. The reflection on dance, its origins, and the value of comparative studies. *Dance Research Annual* 14:99-104.

Yuasa, Y. 1987. *The Body: Toward an Eastern Mind-body Theory*. Albany, New York: State University Press.
Zarrilli, P. 1990. What does it mean to 'become the character": power, presence, and transcendence in Asian in-body disciplines of practice. In Schechner, R. & Appel, L. (Ed.). *By Means of Performance* (pp. 131-148). New York: Cambridge Press.

INDEX

Aesthetic 13, 35, 37, 46, 48-50, 53, 76, 96, 110, 145, 146, 168
Alexander, M. 8, 89
Aragoto 42-44, 50, 87, 104, 145
Asobi 22, 145
Ballet 36, 42, 62, 73, 136
Bioenergetics 9, 89
Blacking, J. 12
Brandon, J. 10, 151
Bunraku 35, 38, 40, 107
Clifford, J. 6
Communication 9, 71, 86, 88, 90, 92, 93, 149, 150, 153, 155-157, 158, 168
Costume 32, 40, 43, 44, 79, 80, 84, 96-98, 99, 100, 101, 105, 109, 125-127, 131, 132, 164, 166
De Vos, G. 157
Duty 82, 88, 90-92, 106, 149, 152, 153, 164, 165 (see also Giri)
Embodied 11, 103
Enryo 153
Fan 37-39, 46, 61, 75, 76, 79, 81, 86, 109, 131
Feldenkrais, M. 8, 89
Fuji 23, 56, 79, 83, 98, 99, 108, 111
Fujima school 19, 23, 25-28, 32, 47, 56, 57, 70, 79, 87, 109, 123, 137, 146, 148-150, 160, 164, 168
Fujinami-kai 2, 4, 7, 28, 57, 61, 66, 69, 70, 99, 122, 125, 128, 134, 135, 136, 141
Furi 37-39, 78, 97
Furisode 97-99
Gaman 153
Geisha 16, 18, 22, 28, 67, 72, 79, 81, 86, 99, 101, 106, 107, 109, 161

Gidayu 41, 103
Giri 88, 92, 106, 155 (see also Duty)
Glenn, E. 26
Graceful 39, 67, 79, 83, 106, 108
Gunji, M. 18, 36-38, 40, 50, 51, 85, 104
Hall, E. 125, 129
Hana 48, 79, 82, 104, 108-110
Henge 44, 98
High Context 155
Hikinuki 98, 138
Hinatsu, Diane 62, 82, 87, 99, 101, 111, 167
Iemoto 19, 21-25, 27, 53, 56, 65, 70, 88, 145, 146, 148-151, 161, 167
Iki 51
Image 42, 75, 77, 105, 107, 109, 121, 163-165
Interethnic 55, 92, 124, 137, 142, 146, 151, 159, 161
Interpersonal 153, 154, 156, 157
Introspection 3, 47
Intuitive 43, 46, 50, 158
Issei 26, 55, 143, 146, 149-151, 159, 161, 168
Izutsu, T. & T. 48, 49, 51
Johnson, M. 7, 8, 45, 53
Kabuki 16-18 19, 22, 23, 25, 28, 32, 35-41, 43, 44, 45, 63, 65, 66, 2, 80, 83, 84, 87, 96-99, 102-104, 105-108, 123, 125, 134, 136-138, 141, 142, 145, 149, 162, 168
Kagura 16, 21, 85, 102
Kakucho 50
Kami 22, 36, 75-77, 100
Kan'emon Fujima 17, 18, 23, 25, 27
Kanji 18, 56, 105
Kansho Fujima 25, 27, 29, 56, 63,

136, 146, 149, 168
Kata 11, 46, 79, 81, 84-88, 92, 105, 108, 109
Kinesthetic 9, 11, 58, 78, 81, 89-91, 110, 143, 152
Kitano, H. L. 153, 166
Kiyomoto 103, 104
Ko-joruri 40, 41
Koken 92, 98, 99, 138
Kominz, Larry 42-44, 65
Kondo, D. 154, 155
Kumadori 101
Kyogen 17, 44, 65
Ma 50, 90, 92
Mai 19, 28, 37, 39, 109, 136, 137
Make-up 25, 40, 70, 92, 96, 100, 101, 125, 126, 132, 136, 141, 142, 146, 164
Malm, W. 103, 104
Marcus, G. 5, 6
Masakazu, Y. 48, 50
Mask 60, 65, 80, 85, 101, 102, 114
Matsu 23, 56, 83, 86, 108
Matsuri 30, 126, 161
Modern dance 36, 62, 134, 136, 167
Multi-cultural 158
Murphy, M. 8, 9
Music 2, 18, 20, 25, 41, 42, 45, 46, 60-62, 72-74, 77, 81, 82, 86, 87, 96, 99, 103, 104, 130, 133, 139-141, 163
Nagauta 99, 103, 104
Natori 15, 23, 28, 29, 56-58, 60, 63, 64, 68, 70, 71, 74, 83, 85-88, 90, 92, 99, 122, 124, 125-127, 131-134, 136, 138, 143, 148-151, 156, 159-161, 167, 168
New Year 30, 31, 43, 70, 107, 109, 140, 142, 161
Ninjo 155
Nisei 26, 55, 132, 143, 146, 150, 154, 158, 159
Noh 16, 19, 35, 37, 40, 44-46, 48-50, 65, 83, 84, 104, 107, 145, 162, 168
Nonverbal 9, 10, 11, 46, 88, 90, 93, 128, 150, 154, 155, 158, 165
Notation 87, 123
Obligation 23, 58, 63, 70, 88, 93, 106, 149, 150, 155 (see also On)
Obon 16, 29, 45, 87, 121, 122, 129, 130-134, 140, 142, 143, 161, 162, 164
Odori 16, 20, 28, 37-39, 45, 61, 64, 78, 81, 97, 100, 101, 104, 126, 130, 131, 133-137, 143, 149, 162
Ogi 38, 106
Okisa 50
Omoiyari 153, 155
On 23, 149, 150 (see also Obligation)
Onnagata 39-44, 63, 98, 145
Ontario 4, 11, 15, 26-32, 55, 58, 60, 67, 70, 73, 74, 86, 121, 122, 129, 130-134, 139-143, 148, 149, 160-162, 164
Ortner, S. 165
Performance 7, 9, 12, 13, 16, 18,

21, 22, 24-26, 35, 36, 38, 39, 44, 50-52, 56, 57, 61, 63, 69, 70, 82, 83, 95, 96, 97, 99, 101, 102-105, 107, 109, 110, 121, 122, 124, 125-129, 131-135, 137-139, 141-143, 146, 148, 152, 153, 160-162, 165
Portland 1, 2, 4, 5, 7, 11, 15, 26-30, 55-59, 61-67, 69, 70, 73, 74, 107, 121, 122, 125, 134-136, 139-143, 148, 149, 159, 160-162, 166, 167
Props 44, 59, 73, 76, 77, 79, 84, 90, 92, 96, 98, 109, 130, 131
Recital 15, 28, 29, 46, 60, 64, 66, 70, 80, 96, 99, 100, 122-125, 127, 128, 132, 136, 141, 142, 149, 162
Rimer, T. 48, 50, 66
Rosaldo, R. 5, 6
Sabi 48
Said, E. 2, 5, 25, 71, 87, 89, 128, 130, 141, 158, 167
Samurai 37, 67, 72, 84, 86, 101, 106, 109, 127, 131, 133
Sansei 55, 71, 146, 154, 159, 161, 168
Schechner, R. 139
Seishin 20, 105, 110, 152, 153
Shamisen 16, 20, 28-30, 39, 40, 45, 60, 73, 103, 104, 135
Shosagoto 17, 39, 44, 45, 83, 87, 98, 99, 103
Snell, Diana 64, 83, 167
Somatic 8, 9, 11, 12, 46, 49-52, 77, 89, 106, 146, 150, 158
Spicer, E. 163, 164
Spokane 15, 27, 28, 55, 56, 70, 121, 122, 134, 136-143, 148, 160, 161, 162, 165, 166
Stroup, Miyoko 28, 30, 59, 68, 70, 100, 114, 115, 125, 134, 136, 149
Su odori 97, 100, 101
Suriashi 37, 84
Symbol 78, 105, 108, 109, 165, 166
Tanabata 121, 134, 135, 140, 161, 162
Teen-ager 31, 71, 76, 80, 86, 126
Theme 79, 81, 99, 108, 109
Tokiwazu 103, 104
Training 5, 7, 9-11, 12, 18, 22, 24, 25, 32, 46, 48-52, 66, 68, 81, 86, 89, 90, 95, 97, 105, 106, 109, 145, 146, 149, 150, 152, 153, 157, 158, 161, 165
Uchi deshi 20, 21, 145
Utsuri 50, 90
Uyesugi, Barbara 2, 4, 5, 28, 30, 57, 66, 68, 70, 73, 80, 100, 101, 112, 124, 128, 134, 136, 137, 149
Wagoto 42, 43, 87
Western theatre 36, 85
Yuasa, Y. 48, 49, 52
Yugen 48-50, 110
Zarrilli, P. 9-11
Zeami 37, 46, 48-52, 145